DIARY OF PRAYERS FOR AUTOIMMUNE DISEASES

NIKITA THOMPSON

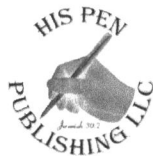

HIS PEN PUBLISHING LLC

The Cataloging-in-Publication Data is on file with the Library of Congress. Printed in the United States of America

Print ISBN: 978-1-944643-39-3
E-Book ISBN: 978-1-944643-40-9
First edition: **2025**

SPECIAL ACKNOWLEDGEMENTS

To my loving husband, Larry Thompson – you are my best friend, my prayer partner, my protector, my forever and always love. Through sickness and health, you stand by my side with grace and strength that inspire me beyond words. I am thankful for your presence in my life, a steadfast pillar of love and devotion. Your commitment to our vows is a testament to the depth of your character. Your words echo with sincerity as you express a desire to bear my pain if only it were possible. I am endlessly grateful for everything you do and for loving me unconditionally amidst life's trials.

To my extraordinary son, DaVante' Thompson - words cannot capture the depth of my admiration for you. When faced with news of my diagnosis, you rose to the occasion with unwavering strength and compassion. Your words became a source of solace, assuring me that brighter days were ahead. Now that you are faced with an uncertain autoimmune condition and Raynaud's phenomenon, your resilience and determination inspire me as you refuse to be defeated by these illnesses. Thank you for embodying encouragement, reliability, empathy, passion, and love as my son. Keep fighting bravely on, my compassionate, generous, dashing, courageous son.

To my astounding daughter, De'Ja Caldwell – you have been a beacon of hope during this most difficult moment in my life. Your continual reinforcement uplifts me every day. In the face of our shared battles of lupus and Raynaud's phenomenon, your strength shines brightly, and your fortitude is awe-inspiring. It is commendable that you took the initiative to educate others as soon as you received your diagnosis; I did not do that. You evolved into a true champion, tackling challenges head-on while promoting awareness by designing and marketing products emphasizing the symptoms of lupus, endometriosis, and Raynaud's phenomenon. My princess, you are a gem. You are magnificent, remarkable, strong, stunning, exceptional, and amazing.

My incredible mother, Mattie Austin – since the moment I received my diagnosis, your unconditional love has been a source of immense strength. Throughout my journey, despite my tears and hardships, you stood by me with an unshakeable heart, witnessing my struggles without faltering. Your aid and selfless nature have truly been recognized and are deeply appreciated. I can't picture how challenging it must have been to deal with all my adventures over the years, but you handled it with grace and patience. How much you mean to me cannot be described adequately in words. I cherish and love you, Mom. I am thankful for your wonderful assistance, beautiful woman.

To my cherished sister, Jamisha Austin - you do not realize how much you stimulate and propel me to be courageous in this new routine. I am reminded of God's presence as I witness your determination not to succumb to lupus and scleroderma without a fight. As I am dealing with the same diseases, I reflect on how you manage them on a daily basis. Your efforts are relentless, and you don't give up. Watching you fight in this battle motivates me and empowers me to continue my own fight with self-confidence. A sister's love is truly one of a kind. I express my heartfelt gratitude for the backing and affection from my incredible, blessed, and tough sister.

To my wonderful lupus survivors group – I express my gratitude for the kindness, support, and love you have extended to me. You are not alone, as we are in the fight together. You are beautiful, strong, unique, loved, blessed, and a joy to be around. You are not a prisoner of this disease. You all are tenacious and can handle whatever Satan brings your way because of your faith in God. You are a living testament, and your experiences will serve as a source of inspiration and blessing for others.

To my unwavering supporters – LaCricia A'ngelle, Karen Billingsley, Dr. Michael Burnette, La'Quan Charity, Andrea Crittle,

Clay/Dorothy Horton, Anicette Richardson, Freda Scott, Misty Smith, Bridgette Stevenson, and Valencia Wright - each of you has a distinct and treasured place in my heart. I want to express my gratitude for your direct firmness, exhorting words, and love. I am thankful for your friendship, positive demeanor, and relentless prompting to rest when I was tempted to exceed my limits. Each of you played, and continue to play, a crucial role in positively impacting my life, whether through your professionalism, kindness, or by offering entertainment during my health challenges and periods of writer's block, often without your awareness. I thank those who contributed by reading, editing, or providing financial support to bring this book to publication.

CONTENTS

FOREWORD

One of the easiest things for me to say is how much I love, admire, and appreciate Nikita. Friend, wife, mother of my children, closest confidant, prayer warrior, and most trusted person in the world are only a few adjectives that come to mind when I think of her. The tangible ways she reveals the gift she is to me, our family, her community, and humanity flow so effortlessly from her. But people might not realize that all those wonderful qualities directly relate to her faith in Jesus Christ.

I have witnessed her faith in Christ for the last 40 years of our lives together. Her faith in Christ has been a continuous growth process. She has blossomed into an amazing spirit. Just when you think you have a box to fit her in, she transforms into someone more wonderful than the last.

As youth, Nikita and I were like two starry-eyed kids. She was, and is, one of the most beautiful and amazing women that has EVER crossed my life. Her beauty radiates from her spirit and reflects in how she presents herself to others. She loves people tenaciously.

When this disease attacked her, she did not lose hope. There were days she rejected the diagnosis. She began to declare her victory, even as the signs, symptoms, and fight intensified. One of the things I admire about her is that even when she had thoughts of "why me," she immediately declared, "Because God knows I will fight!"

She has no idea just how impressive she is in my eyes. When those early days became very challenging, she would push harder. I would try to convince her to slow down, and she would reply, "I'm going to live like I am living." Each time, I would watch her lean a lot more on God. Some people suffer these attacks and pull back from God, but not Nikita. She has the attitude and spirit of Job housed in a woman's body.

Her strategy is simple. She responds with the weapons she has used for years: prayer, fasting, speaking life over herself, and when necessary, she pours out her tears with complete confidence in God's promise to bottle them up.

When she decided to write this book, she battled against attacks from all areas, including her health, time, confidence in her ability, fatigue, and that nasty foul spirit of doubt. Writing this book was a great opportunity to share her victory over the years she has walked through this journey.

To quote one of her favorite sayings, "If I must go through this, Lord, you get the glory and let my fight be a blessing for someone, somewhere." So, if you are reading this, just know she is here... fasting, praying, declaring her victory, and YOURS! So, you stand strong in the power of God's might. "We all have our faith journey, but in faith, we are never alone."

Prayers of healing to you,
Nikita's Husband

MY STORY

First and foremost, I thank God, for He is my "Rock, my Fortress, and the One who rescues me; My God, my Rock and Strength in whom I trust and take refuge; My Shield, and the Horn of my Salvation, my High Tower—my Stronghold." Psalms 18:2 AMP

This book was written to provide hope to individuals living with autoimmune diseases. I want to emphasize that you are not alone in this struggle. Together, we are warriors on the same battlefield, collectively confronting these relentless diseases that will not defeat us. I must confess that I have, at times, contemplated giving up. However, if I had taken that route, I would not be here to share my insights into your struggles. Numerous days and nights have passed during which my pillows have absorbed my quiet tears, the interior of my vehicle has borne witness to my prayers, and the walls of my home have contained the echoes of my cries directed towards my heavenly Father.

My journey to write this book was fraught with numerous challenges, including fatigue, flare-ups, hospital visits, infections, pain, medical procedures, surgeries, and work obligations. Despite these difficulties, I was aware that this book could be of great help to someone, which inspired me to see it through to completion. Although I wish to be free from pain and affliction of these serious illnesses, I take comfort in knowing that my struggles can benefit others. Until the signs and symptoms of *mixed connective tissue disease* (MCTD) are taken away, I quote healing scriptures daily, drawing strength from my faith in God's promise of restoration. Engaging in daily recitation of healing scriptures led to my healing from protein leakage in my urine, a clear manifestation of God's intervention. I welcome you to join me in a challenge. The challenge is to recite a healing scripture found at the end of the book or to affirm a positive statement at least twice daily for 30 days and see what God can do for you.

Here is my story of how this warrior dealt with and still deals with an autoimmune disease. Without God, I would not have been able to fight this battle. I would have given up a long time ago. Also, while fighting this battle, I am thankful that God has placed the right people in my life. Now, let me take you through my journey.

MY MISDIAGNOSIS

About a year after I married my amazing, handsome, and supportive husband, Larry, I started noticing my fingers would swell for no reason. I went to the doctor, who told me it could be water weight and to stop putting extra salt on my food. He told me to take the diuretic pills that he prescribed and come back in a few weeks.

I took the diuretic pills. They didn't do much for my fingers and nothing for my weight. At my follow-up appointment, the doctor had me discontinue the pills and insisted there was nothing wrong. He stressed that I stay away from salt. Weeks passed, and my fingers finally went back to normal on their own.

My family and I moved from New Jersey to Georgia in 1996 to raise our children in a better environment than what my husband and I grew up in. It was my second year living in Georgia when the swelling started again. I noticed my fingers, feet, and ankles would begin to swell while I was doing my daughter's hair. I did nothing about it at the time.

After a few months of dealing with it, I made an appointment with a new primary physician and explained what was happening and what the physician in New Jersey had stated. To my surprise, he said the same thing the physician in New Jersey said, "take diuretic pills." I informed the physician that when I was prescribed those pills by the previous physician, there was no improvement in my condition. Considering my experience, I chose to refrain from using them. Once again, the swelling disappeared, but it started to come and go more often.

In 2002, my family and I moved to Florida. One day at work, I started feeling sick. I was running a fever and vomiting, and my fingers were cold and hurting severely. I went to the walk-in clinic and was told I had the flu or food poisoning.

My fingers were still hurting after the flu or whatever it was passed. They turned blue, white, and then red once they got warm. All along, my fingers were still swollen, and there was still no diagnosis of what it was or what was causing it. I believe I started showing signs and symptoms of an autoimmune disease in New Jersey and Georgia, but the physicians couldn't diagnose it because it wasn't as popular as it is now.

MY LUPUS DIAGNOSIS

I went to my new primary physician in Florida. "It sounds like you may have lupus, but I am not going to say you have it until the test results come back." When the results confirmed it, my primary physician called and instructed me to see a rheumatologist as soon as possible so I could be treated with the proper medication. At my first visit with the rheumatologist, he took 20 tubes of blood without knowing what was wrong. After the results came back, he still didn't know what was wrong with me, all while my fingers were turning blue and white in front of him.

I was disappointed and mad at the same time. All I could do was cry out to God. I went back to my primary physician and told her what the rheumatologist said. She responded, "What does he mean he doesn't know what's wrong with you? Is he waiting for your fingers to

3

fall off to be able to give you a diagnosis? Can't he see that your fingers are blue?"

As a result, she sent me to Dr. Michael Burnette (who I think is the best in my area). During this visit, I was told I had lupus. When he looked at my hands, he said I also had Raynaud's phenomenon. Additional bloodwork confirmed his diagnosis.

MY CHALLENGES POST-DIAGNOSIS

When I received the results, I was emotional. I thought I was going to die early and not see my children grow up to become adults. I started withdrawing from my husband as well as other people. When I experienced pain in my fingers, I would not say anything to my husband. I thought, *why say anything*? He couldn't take the pain away, and he couldn't stop me from dying. So, I kept the pain to myself and struggled in silence. Low key, I was depressed.

During this time, I was still working with swelling and painful fingers. While working, I observed a sore on my fingertip. I decided to make an appointment with my rheumatologist. Upon examination, he informed me that the sore was referred to as a digital ulcer. The digital ulcer was infected, and the healing process was expected to take several weeks. My job required me to process a lot of paperwork. To avoid any further damage to my finger, he put me on short-term disability, which turned into long-term disability, due to the length of time it took the infection to go away.

Unfortunately, while I was on long-term disability, my job let me go because they could not hold my position any longer. They offered me the opportunity to come back and apply for a different position after I recovered. This was devastating news because I had never been dismissed from a job. I thought, *what kind of nonsense is this, and who made up this crazy rule?* Once I got well, I chose not to apply for another position at that company. I decided to become a Medical Assistant, so I went to school to pursue it.

MY CAREER SHIFT

While I was attending school, my fingers still turned white and blue. They also became numb and painful because it was extremely cold in the building. Whenever I had to practice on others and when I had to take my clinical, it was difficult for me to draw blood and feel for a pulse with cold hands. Dr. Burnette, my rheumatologist, gave me a letter to be excused from getting my blood drawn and getting my finger pricked, as I was at high risk for infections. I thought I would fail my classes because my fingers would stay cold, numb, and painful.

In addition to experiencing cold, numbness, and painful fingers, I was also battling hair loss. I was so emotional and embarrassed when I saw the bald spots on my scalp. I felt like everyone in my class could see them. I purchased a wig and wore it until my hair grew back.

Glory and praises go to God because I graduated with honors. After I graduated and started my internship, I began to have muscle and joint aches and pain appear out of nowhere. I was prescribed ibuprofen. Ibuprofen worked for a while, and then it stopped working. After seeing the rheumatologist for three years, he wanted me to participate in a drug trial program.

MY DRUG TRIAL EXPERIENCE

I decided to participate in the drug trial program. I went for the consultation, and the program was explained to me. I told the nurse I did not want to be a guinea pig. She assured me that everything would be fine. After thinking it over and praying, I said yes to the drug trial.

Anicette was the name of my assigned nurse. She always went out of her way to help me. On one occasion, I saw her at a lupus walk. I told her I was battling another infection. She pulled out her phone and called my rheumatologist right then and there. She told him what was happening and asked him to call in some antibiotics for me. Now, that's what I call a great nurse who went above and beyond her job responsibilities.

While on the trial, Anicette told me she thought I was on the drug

Benlysta and not a placebo. She was right. I was actually on Benlysta before the FDA approved it. I did not feel a big difference physically, but my blood numbers were good. When I finished the trial, I was put on another drug. It didn't work so well, and I had to get off that drug early. My rheumatologist kept me on my regular medications, which include Procardia, Plaquenil, and aspirin, which I still take.

Anicette has been here for me from the beginning stage of my lupus diagnosis, and she is still here for me long after the drug research trial. I called Anicette my personal nurse and counselor then, but now I call her *family*.

MY MEDICAL EMERGENCY

In December 2011, I couldn't breathe, and when I lay down on my left side, it hurt badly. I called my physician and told her what was going on. She called the hospital registration office to have me admitted. When I got to the hospital, they had a bed ready for me. Around the fourth day of my hospital stay, I was not getting any better. I was gasping for air and sleeping a lot, even when I wasn't in pain.

The physician on duty that day told me they ran every test they could, but they could not find what was causing me to feel the way I was feeling. They gave me one last test. Well, that was the proper test. The results came back that I had multiple blood clots in my lungs. Now, the physician could determine the best treatment plan for me.

Each day, I had a different physician check on me to see how well I was doing on the medication. As they walked in, they would say things like, "Hello, beautiful or Hello, sunshine." I never thought to ask them why they called me that. I asked the nurse, and she said, "Because we thought we were going to lose you. Had we known that you had blood clots when you were admitted, you would have gone straight to the ICU."

When I was able to get out of bed on my own, I looked in the mirror and remembered that God had me read the first few chapters of the book of Job a few weeks before being hospitalized. I thought to myself, *why did God have me reread Job?* As I was looking in the mirror and brushing my teeth, I heard, "I had you read Job because I wanted you to know that I gave Satan permission to try you, but he could not kill you." After hearing that, I thanked and praised God. He had protected me and kept angels encamped around me the whole 14 days I was hospitalized. He is still protecting me to this day.

MY NEW DIAGNOSIS

In 2013, I had an official diagnosis of **mixed connective tissue disease (MCTD)**, which consists of **lupus, scleroderma, Raynaud's phenomenon, and Sjögren's Disease**. This is when I first experienced a flare-up. I had no clue what that meant until I was diagnosed with MCTD.

The flare-ups were horrible. The pain was unbearable, and the fatigue was the hardest thing to deal with. I was so exhausted when it was time to go out with family and friends, but I would suck it up and go. Otherwise, I would have slept my life away and didn't want to do that. It was hard for me, as I was battling a lot of pain and shedding a lot of tears.

MY EPIPHANY

There were a lot of days I called on God, asking Him to take away the pain and this disease. I got to the point and finally asked God, "Why me? What did I do to deserve this? There are people out there who have not accepted Jesus Christ as their Savior. They are doing a lot of bad things, and they are not sick. Here I am, trying to live right, but I'm sick and in a lot of pain."

Once I stopped pitying myself, I said, why not me? I have been told that I am strong, and if I am going through something, it doesn't show because I hide it well. I told myself, *you got this*, and God is with you no matter what. He will never leave you nor forsake you. Having a pep talk with myself got me to the point of not going into full depression. Focusing and trusting in God and His word was how I went through life with my new normal, even though I know God is healing me.

MY LUPUS SUPPORT GROUP

A friend, Karen Billingsley, told me years ago that I would have a lupus support group. I replied, "No, I won't." She would bring it up as time passed, and my response was always the same. Once again, another person in my life was right.

2018 I started a lupus support group called Lupus Survivor, Inc. 2022 the government officially recognized our group as a nonprofit 501c3 organization. This group was formed so that everyone who came in contact with us would know that they were not alone and that we were all fighting this battle together. I mentioned often in the support group that we all may have the same diseases, but our symptoms are different, just like butterflies come in various shapes and sizes. There are no two butterflies alike.

I take great pride in having a loyal core team that has been with me since the inception. The recent integration of new members has officially converted our group into a co-ed team. Without these great people, I would lack a support group. No complaining is allowed in the group. Complaining will get us nowhere! So, we leave the disease(s) at the door and have fun. We don't talk about dying. We talk about living life and enjoying it to the fullest.

The group aims to bring awareness to autoimmune diseases through our annual *Lupus Ball* and the *Invisible and Visible Autoimmune Diseases Walk*. Our goal is to help fellow autoimmune disease warriors. We launched these successful events in 2023. At the walk, we ask for donations of school supplies so that we can give them to the local schools in need.

Also, our group has a talented male warrior as well. While he is battling an autoimmune disease, he still manages to capture all the work we do. He is our photographer, videographer, and designer.

MY BATTLE CONTINUES

Fast forward to now. I am still battling with a lot of pain. I feel like the pain is normal for me now. I have been struggling with back, hip, shoulder, and foot pain over the past few years. I am at high risk of getting infections in my fingers with Raynaud's phenomenon. In 2023, I was hospitalized for osteomyelitis (infection in the bone) in my finger.

I feel like I'm in a war battling against myself. The brain fog is real, and the fatigue is the worst. I tell myself, "I shall not die but live and declare the works of the Lord."

I go to bed late now, not because I want to, but because I can't sleep. Then I find myself getting up late in the morning. My wonderful husband tells me to sleep and not worry about the house or cooking; he will bring something home for us. My son suggests I nap during the day, and my daughter advises me to rest. I don't listen well, and I push and push until I can't do it any longer.

MY CHILDREN'S DIAGNOSES

As I write this portion about my children, I am in tears. While I am battling to make sure I'm present and available for my family, I found out that my children have autoimmune diseases. My daughter was diagnosed with endometriosis, discoid lupus, Raynaud's phenomenon, and systemic lupus. My son was diagnosed with an unpredictable autoimmune disease and Raynaud's phenomenon.

At first, it was hard to hear about my children having these autoimmune diseases. When I found out about the results, I held back my tears so I wouldn't break down in front of them. When my children were not around, I cried to God and let my tears be my prayer. Once I got past the tears, I prayed that God would be with them, heal them, and take away their pain. No parent wants to see their child (children) in pain, knowing they can't do anything to help them. I wished their sickness upon myself so they would not have to go through it.

My son doesn't want to tell people about the diseases he's battling because he doesn't want anyone to have pity on him. I told my son that what he feels is what he feels. No one can tell him how his body feels. I told him everyone with an autoimmune disease does not experience the same symptoms. I reminded him that he has to go through the process just like everyone else has to go through their process.

I make sure I'm available to go to their doctor's appointments. When or if they don't know the questions to ask, I can ask for them. My children will not fight this battle alone as long as I live. We are in this fight together!

When I was first diagnosed, I was told that lupus, scleroderma, and Raynaud's disease were not hereditary. However, physicians now say that they are. Not only do my children and I have it, but my mother and my sister were diagnosed with it as well. My family and I are strong. We will fight the battle until we cannot fight anymore.

MY HOPE

Honestly, I am only surviving and have not given up because of my Heavenly Father, Jehovah Rapha, my Healer. I will leave you with this saying that I use for my support group and myself, along with scriptures that help me get through tough times until the manifestation of my healing comes:

"I live like I am living and not like I am sick."

2 KINGS 20:5 (NKJV)

"Return and tell Hezekiah, the leader of My people, 'Thus says the Lord, the God of David your father: "I have heard your prayer, I have seen your tears; surely, I will heal you. On the third day, you shall go up to the house of the Lord."

2 CORINTHIANS 1:3-4 (AMPC)

"Blessed be the God and Father of our Lord Jesus Christ, the Father of sympathy (pity and mercy) and the God [Who is the Source] of every comfort (consolation and encouragement), Who comforts (consoles and encourages) us in every trouble (calamity and affliction), so that we may also be able to comfort (console and encourage) those who are in any kind of trouble or distress, with the comfort (consolation and encouragement) with which we are comforted (consoled and encouraged) by God."

2 Corinthians [12:9 MSG]

Once I heard that, I was glad to let it happen. I quit focusing on the handicap and began appreciating the gift. It was a case of Christ's strength moving in on my weakness. Now I take limitations in stride, and with good cheer, these limitations that cut me down to size— abuse, accidents, opposition, bad breaks. I just let Christ take over! And so, the weaker I get, the stronger I become.

LUPUS SURVIVORS' TESTIMONIES

TESTIMONY #1

I WAS DIAGNOSED with lupus at the age of 65. I was having a problem with my arm and hand. I would get up with my arms hurting and my hands and fingers numb. By mid-morning, I had no aches, pain, or numbness in my arms and hands. This went on for a few days. I thought I was having a heart attack or stroke. Finally, I went to the doctor and told her what was going on. Because of the autoimmune history in my family, she sent me for tests. Two days later, the test results came back that I was positive for lupus.

I explained to my doctor that I had two spine surgeries and that the neurosurgeon had put me on steroids. Also, I advised her that the neurosurgeon sent the samples of what they took off my spine and sent them to a spine and scleroderma specialist and major labs. I had no signs of lupus or scleroderma at the time, and the results came back negative. My primary physician also explained that because I had been taking steroids for so long, the steroids were masking the lupus.

Ultimately, I don't know how long I have actually had lupus. I'm experiencing upper and lower back pain, tingling in my fingers, and hand pain, with one finger having extreme pain in it, along with it being hard to move for minutes. Both of my hands get so cold that they become numb. My legs and feet feel like I have been sitting in a bucket of ice. The pain is real, and the struggle is real. Every day I wake up, I don't know how I will feel.

Mattie Austin –
Lupus Survivor

TESTIMONY #2

WHEN I THINK of sharing my journey, I often get stuck at "Where do I begin?" There's so much to say about my experience that I'm unsure how to consolidate it into a few paragraphs. But I will take you down the events that have gotten me here, starting with March 2020.

One morning, I was getting ready for church, and while brushing my hair, I noticed a bald spot a little larger than a quarter. I immediately panicked. I sought out help from my primary care physician. She diagnosed me with a fungal infection of the scalp (ringworm). I was put on antibiotics. The severe itchiness that came with the spot led me to Google. I found out that apple cider vinegar has antibacterial and antifungal properties, which can help with infections in the scalp. I applied that for about a week and saw a big turnaround. My hair was even growing back.

Fast forward to December 2020. The bald spot that was once the size of a quarter had tripled in size. I also developed two other bald spots. I contacted my PCP again. She wanted to give me another round of antibiotics. I knew in my heart that this couldn't be an infection, so I declined the antibiotics and decided to see a dermatologist.

January 2021. I had laparoscopic surgery to discover if I had endometriosis. During my recovery, I started feeling a long list of symptoms I had never experienced. I contacted my gynecologist, who stated what I felt was unrelated to the surgery.

Toward the end of my recovery, I went to have my scalp examined by a dermatologist. The dermatologist looked at my scalp for less than thirty seconds before saying, "This is not an infection. This looks like an autoimmune response." I freaked out silently while she went on to say she believed I had discoid lupus. She also stated I would need to get bloodwork done, as well as a biopsy, for her to diagnose me accurately.

In between getting my labs completed, I visited her again for a follow-up on the treatment she prescribed. During that visit, she wanted to do an ANA test to rule out systemic lupus. About a week later, I received a call from the doctor saying that my results were in. She suggested I see a rheumatologist.

February 2021. I had my first appointment with a rheumatologist. During that appointment, she stated that she was 80% to 90% sure that I had systemic lupus. She would know for certain once my bloodwork came back. Fast forward to March 2021, I had been diagnosed with endometriosis, discoid lupus, systemic lupus, and Raynaud's. I was completely floored. The only thing that kept me from losing my mind was my faith in God and knowing that if my mom could make it, so could I. Also, I had already been involved in the Lupus Survivor group pre-diagnosis, so I knew the ladies would support me post-diagnosis.

I spent 13 years dealing with horrifying menstrual cycles and went to three different gynecologists before getting a diagnosis. I also went a little over a year being misdiagnosed with a fungal infection that really was an autoimmune disease, which resulted in me losing hair and developing scarring on my scalp in multiple areas of my head. I want my story to empower you to advocate for yourself relentlessly until you get the correct answers and treatments.

Remember, no matter how lonely it feels, you are not alone. God hears and bottles up every tear you cry with the intention to repay you with joy.

"My flesh and my heart may fail, but God is the strength of my heart and my portion forever." Psalm 73:26 ESV

De'Ja Caldwell –
Endometriosis and Lupus Survivor

TESTIMONY #3

My journey began a little over 17 years ago when I was diagnosed with SLE, better known as lupus. After my diagnosis, my first thoughts were, *finally someone believes me,* immediately followed by, *I'm only 23. Will I be on medication for the rest of my life?* At that point in my life, I felt like a guinea pig, but what choice did I have? I could either be on medication for the rest of my life and live a somewhat normal life, or refuse treatment and possibly die.

Again, I was only 23…I wanted to live, so I chose to do just that. After much prayer (because God knows His strength was what kept me moving forward), I was placed in a blind trial study group for those with lupus, which in return saved my life and put me in remission for several years. I could move without hurting; my feet weren't swollen, and I could finally live like I did before. Life had given me another chance.

Fast forward to 2020. Lupus returned as though it were trying to make up for lost time. Joint pains were more severe and now present in my wrists and hands, making it difficult to do everyday tasks. I can recall one moment when I couldn't even remove my contacts…that was a sad day. But of course, I couldn't allow lupus to win. So, I cried a bit, got back up, put my gloves on, and got back in the ring. I was ready to fight again.

I now had a little girl who looked at me as though I were superwoman. She still does, so I couldn't let her or myself wallow in my pain. I had to fight. Besides, I had just the right people in my corner to help with my recovery, which included my lupus support group. I often tell people that it's one thing to discuss your illness with someone without lupus and hope they understand, but it's another thing to talk about it with a group of people who have experienced what you have. There's comfort in knowing that you're not alone. Prayer, faith, listening to my body, self-care, and surrounding myself with people who genuinely want to see me at my highest level of life are what have gotten me this far.

To all my newly diagnosed *Lupies*, lupus is tough, but baby, you're tougher. You've got this!

Guerdy Jean Gaines –
Lupus Survivor

TESTIMONY #4

LIVING with lupus is not easy. It breaks you down so you can rebuild yourself piece by piece. We face daily battles against pain, fatigue, and uncertainty about what the future holds. Yet, during these struggles, I am constantly holding on and sustained by the grace of God and the fighter spirit he put inside of me.

I know firsthand the toll that lupus can take on our bodies, minds, and spirits. At times, you may want to give up. You may feel alone, like there's an alien inside your body that you have no control over. But little by little, you will learn how to accommodate yourself in this new reality of survival mode. It's a journey filled with ups and downs, triumphs, and setbacks. At my hardest times, when I was in excruciating pain, I felt like I was hopeless. My mother used to pray for me and tell me that God was in control. Brushing her fingers around my hair, I would reply in an angry but cheerful way, "Please tell God to pass the control so I can change this channel. "She would laugh, making a tragic comedy of the circumstances. Finding laughter can be therapeutic. Learning to laugh about our situation can help us handle the pain better.

Through all my experiences, I am determined to keep pushing forward, one day at a time. Having a support system of family members, friends, and lupus groups is very important, but mainly, having hope in God to get me through this is the main reason I'm still here. Knowing that even though I have lupus, it does not define who I am as a person. Being part of this support group is a blessing. Having other *lupies* that I can relate to is very important to me. Before the group, I used to feel alone and estranged in my body. I could not relate to anyone. No one understood me, not even my family, who were close to me and saw my changes.

Within the group, I could talk freely about my symptoms without judgment. This support made it easier for me to understand what I was experiencing, that I wasn't alone, and that others faced similar challenges at different stages. This helped me work around my struggles with an open mind.

I'm thankful for everyone who contributes to my life and helps me, whether by listening to me, giving advice, or praying. The support group is my family, full of wisdom and resilience. I admire each one of them. Their strength gives me hope.

No matter how tough the road may seem, we have the strength within us to overcome any obstacle that comes our way. Let us continue to lift each other up, support each other through the good days and the bad, and remind ourselves that even in the darkest moments, there is always a glimmer of hope shining through.

With love & support,
Diery L Arias
Lupus Survivor
Conditions: lupus, subtumor cerebri, arthritis, neuropathy, hypothyroidism, anxiety, and depression
Top of Form – Feeling as well as possible
When in pain, I read: Psalms 6

DIARY OF PRAYERS FOR AUTOIMMUNE DISEASES

ADDISON'S DISEASE

REJOICE IN THE LORD, O you righteous! For praise from the upright is beautiful. Oh, how great is Your goodness, which You have laid up for those who fear You, which You have prepared for those who trust in You in the presence of the sons of men! You do great things and unsearchable, marvelous things without number. Thank You, Father, in advance for answering me before I call to You. According to Your Word, while I am still speaking to You about my needs, You will hear my prayers!

I express to you my concerns regarding this hormonal disorder. I request that you touch my body so that my adrenal glands may produce an appropriate quantity of cortisol and aldosterone, Father. This condition is making me feel sick, causing diarrhea, vomiting, and a lack of appetite, which is leading to weight loss. Decrease and eliminate the pain in my muscles, joints, and abdomen. Increase my blood pressure so that I will not faint, especially when I am alone. Father, increase my low blood glucose so that I won't experience blurred vision, difficulty concentrating, slurred speech, confused thinking, numbness, or worse, have a seizure or go into a coma. I am extremely fatigued daily, and I am asking for strength, energy, and recharging so that I can perform my daily tasks.

Your Word states that You give power to the weak, and to those who have no might, You increase strength. I thank You in advance for healing, strength, and restoration. I decree and declare that my urinary, musculoskeletal, immune, circulatory, integumentary, and digestive systems, along with my hormone-secreting, blood, and immune system cells, will be in harmony with the design You established for their functionality.

According to Your Word, Jesus was wounded for my transgressions, He was bruised for my iniquities, and the chastisement of my peace was upon Him, and by His stripes, **I AM HEALED!**

Death and life are in the power of the tongue, so I speak life over my body. I decree and declare prosperity of healing over my body, in Jesus' name. Whatever medication(s) I am prescribed, I pray that I will not have any side effects and it will help me, not further harm me, in the name of Jesus. Thank You for restoring my health and rejuvenating me, for You are the source of all healing. Father, thank You for hearing the effectual, fervent prayer of a righteous man/woman. You are the All-Knowing and All-Powerful God, who I love dearly. Amen!

{Psalm 33:1, Psalm 31:19, Job 5:9, Isaiah 65:24 (TLB), Isaiah 40:29, Job 22:28, Isaiah 53:5, Proverbs 18:21, 3 John 2, Jeremiah 30:17, James 5:16b, Romans 11:33, Jeremiah 32:17} NKJV

ALOPECIA AREATA

Father, I clap my hands and shout to You with the voice of triumph. I sing praises to You, God, praises to my King. For You are the King of all the earth. I sing to You a psalm of praise. You reign over the nations and sit on Your holy throne. God, You are my refuge and strength, a very present help in trouble.

I will praise You, for I am fearfully and wonderfully made; marvelous are Your works, and that my soul knows very well. I cast my cares, [anxieties, worries, and concerns], once and for all, on You, for You care about me [with deepest affection] and watch over me very carefully.

I humbly come before You asking for healing and restoration from sudden hair loss on my scalp, face, and other body parts. This hair loss has brought on unwanted tears because of this sudden life change. Father, I ask that You stop my immune system from targeting my hair follicles so that thinning, falling out, and formation of bald spots will cease. Strengthen and restore my hair follicles so that my hair can grow back stronger, healthier, fuller, and prettier than before. I pray that my hair loss is temporary and not permanent.

I thank You, Father, for being with me during this stressful time. I know that I can count on You to be by my side and to comfort me. Thank You, Father, that You have heard my prayer, You have seen my tears. Surely, You will heal me. I decree and declare my integumentary system, along with my blood and immune system cells, will be in harmony with the design You established for their functionality. Your Word says that Jesus was wounded for my transgressions, He was bruised for my iniquities; the chastisement of my peace was upon Him, and by His stripes, **I AM HEALED!**

Death and life are in the power of the tongue, so I speak life over my body. I decree and declare prosperity of healing over my body. In Jesus' name. Whatever medication(s) I am prescribed, I pray that I will not have any side effects and it will help me, not further harm me, in the name of Jesus. While I am waiting for my hair to grow back, help me to continue to trust, be patient, and lean on You, Father. I thank You that my healing shall spring forth speedily. Father, thank You for being my Comforter. Amen!

{Psalm 47:1, Psalm 47:6-8, Psalm 46:1, Psalm 139:14, 1 Peter 5:17 (AMP), 2 Kings 20:5, Job 22:28, Isaiah 53:5, Proverbs 18:21, 3 John 2, Isaiah 58:8a, 2 Corinthians 1:3-4} NKJV

ANKYLOSING SPONDYLITIS

I will praise and give thanks to You, O Lord, among the people; I will sing praises to You among the nations. For Your faithfulness and lovingkindness are great, reaching to the heavens, and Your truth to the clouds. Be exalted above the heavens, O God; let Your glory and majesty be over all the earth. From the end of the earth, I will sing praises; You God are my strength, I will sing praises; For You God are my stronghold (my refuge, my protector, my high tower), the God who shows me (steadfast) lovingkindness. Father, my body is the temple of the Holy Spirit. I am not my own. I am Your masterpiece.

You have created me anew in Christ Jesus, so I can do the good things You planned for me long ago. Satan, I am giving you notice and exercising the authority and power granted by God to trample upon serpents and scorpions, and over all the power of the enemy, and nothing shall in any way harm me. I will not be ignorant of any of your devices. Satan, you are a liar! I will enjoy life, and have it in abundance (to the full, till it overflows).

Satan, I am a warrior. I serve a Mighty Good God who can heal any sickness and disease. Father, smother and release the inflammation in my spinal joints so that I will not continue to have discomfort and chronic pain. Decrease and eliminate the pain and stiffness that I am having in my hips, heels, ribs, lower back, buttocks, shoulders, and small joints of my hands and feet. Give me strength and energy in my body when I am battling fatigue. Please do not let my eyes, heart, and lungs get affected by this disease, Father.

When I decree a thing, it shall be established unto me, and the light shall shine upon my ways. I decree and declare that my nervous, respiratory, and skeletal systems, along with my blood and immune system cells, will be in harmony with the design You established for their functionality.

According to Your Word, Jesus was wounded for my transgressions, He was bruised for my iniquities, and the chastisement of my peace was upon Him, and by His stripes, **I AM HEALED!** Death and life are in the power of the tongue, so I speak life over my body. I decree and declare prosperity of healing over my body. In Jesus' name.

Whatever medication(s) I am prescribed, I pray that I will not have any side effects and it will help me, not further harm me, in the name

of Jesus. Blessed to be in the land, I'm free from the enemy's worries. Whenever I'm sick and in bed, God becomes my nurse and nurses me back to health. Father, You do not forget to help me when I am in pain. You do not turn away from me, the one who suffered. When I call to You, God, for help, You answer my prayer. Thank You for being the Good Shepherd. Amen!

{Psalm 57:9-11 (AMP), Psalm 59:17 (AMP), 1 Corinthians 6:19, Ephesians 2:10 (NLT), Luke 10:19 (AMPC), 2 Corinthians 2:11, Job 22:28, Isaiah 53:5, Proverbs 18:21, 3 John 2, Psalm 91:3 (MSG), Psalm 22:24 (EASY), John 10:11} NKJV

ANTIPHOSPHOLIPID ANTIBODY SYNDROME

Father, because Your loving-kindness is better than life, my lips shall praise You. Thus, I will bless You while I live; I will lift up my hands in Your name. Let my mouth be filled with Your praise and with Your glory all day. I will hope continually and will praise You yet more and more.

I come boldly to the throne of grace that I may obtain mercy and find grace to help in a time of need. Father, I come before You humbly asking that You touch my immune system and stop it from attacking itself and causing abnormal blood clots to form. Decrease and dissolve any blood clots that I have. Relieve my skin of rashes, Father. So, I ask that You clear it up. Touch my body so that I won't have any unexpected problems like a stroke or heart attack.

Thank You for not letting any illness kill me. I decree and declare that my cardiovascular, integumentary, immune, and respiratory systems, along with my blood and immune cells, will be in harmony with the design You established for their functionality.

According to Your word, Jesus was wounded for my transgressions, He was bruised for my iniquities, and the chastisement of my peace was upon Him, and by His stripes, **I AM HEALED!** Death and life are in the power of the tongue, so I speak life over my body. I decree and declare prosperity of healing over my body. In Jesus' name.

Whatever medication(s) I am prescribed, I pray that I will not have any side effects and it will help me, not further harm me, in the name of Jesus. Thank You, Father, that You are the source of all healing, for You are the All-knowing Physician, Jehovah Rapha (The Lord Who Heals). Amen!

FOR THOSE WHO ARE PREGNANT

I pray that You protect my womb and protect my seed so that I will not have a miscarriage or a stillborn. Father, I ask that You touch my womb and allow me to carry my baby full-term without complications. Your word states that I am to bear fruit, reproduce, lavish life on the earth, and live bountifully. When I serve You, Father, You will bless my food and water. Thank You, Father, that You will get rid of the sickness among me, and there won't be any miscarriages nor barren women in my land. You will make sure I live a full and complete life. Thank You, Father, for keeping me safe so that no trap will catch me. Amen!

{Psalm 63:3-4, Psalm 71:8, Psalm 71:14, Hebrews 4:16, Genesis 9:7 (MSG), Exodus 23:25-26 (MSG), Psalm 91:3 (EASY), Job 22:28, Isaiah 53:5, Proverbs 18:21, 3 John 2, Romans 3:11, Matthew 9:12, Exodus 15:26} NKJV

If you continue to experience chest pains, please go to the hospital or call 911.

AUTOIMMUNE HEPATITIS

Father, I will sing to You as long as I live; I will sing praise to You, my God, while I have my being. I will shout joyfully to You, Lord, and break forth in song, rejoice, and sing praises. I give thanks to You, Lord, for You are good! For Your mercy endures forever. The Spirit of God has made me. The breath of the Almighty gives me life. I praise You with all that is in me, Father.

I thank You, God, for everything. No matter the circumstances, I am grateful and give thanks, for this is Your will, God, for me (who is) in Christ Jesus (the Revealer and Mediator of that will). Father, I am seeking help in a time of need. I ask that You decrease and relieve the pain I'm experiencing in my joints, muscles, and abdomen. Smother and release the inflammation in my liver so that my immune system will stop attacking my liver cells. Soothe my itchy skin and take away the jaundice and rashes.

Decrease and eliminate the symptoms of nausea, loss of appetite, dark urine, absence of menses, and/or pale stools. Decrease and reverse my enlarged liver, Father, so my liver can heal. Protect my liver from being further damaged so that it will not lead to cirrhosis or liver failure. I pray that You give my hepatologist and gastroenterologist wisdom and knowledge on the best treatment plan for me.

Father, I come to You with faith, not doubting that You can and will heal me from this disease. For You will restore my health and heal my wounds. Satan, you are on notice that I cancel any assignments you have on my life. Anything that came from you, Satan, does not belong to me, but HEALING DOES! Jesus went about all the cities and villages to not only teach and preach the gospel but to heal every sickness and every disease among the people. Father, if You can heal them, I know that You can heal me as well because there is no partiality with You, God.

I decree and declare that my digestive, integumentary, and urinary systems, along with my blood and immune system cells, will be in harmony with the design You established for their functionality.

According to Your Word, Jesus was wounded for my transgressions, He was bruised for my iniquities, and the chastisement of my peace was upon Him, and by His stripes, **I AM HEALED!** Death and life are in the power of the tongue, so I speak life over my body. I decree and declare prosperity of healing over my body. In Jesus' name.

Whatever medication(s) I am prescribed, I pray that I will not have any side effects and it will help me, not further harm me, in the name of Jesus. God, You are not a man, You do not lie. You are not human, and You do not change Your mind. You have spoken and have not failed me. You make good on Your promises. Thank You that Your word will not return void, but it shall accomplish what You please. Thank You for being The Author and The Finisher of my faith, Father. Amen!

{Psalm 104:33, Psalm 98:4, Psalm 107:1, Job 33:4, 1 Thessalonians 5:18m (AMPC), Jeremiah 30:17, Matthew 4:23, Romans 2:11, Job 22:28, Isaiah 53:5, Proverbs 18:21, 3 John 2, Isaiah 55:11, Numbers 23:19 (NLT), Hebrews 12:2} NKJV

AUTOIMMUNE INNER EAR DISEASE (AIED)

I want to lift up Your holy name and give praises to You before I ask anything from You. Lord, I worship and exalt You! For You, Lord, my God, are holy. I praise You, Father, for Your great love and for the wonderful things You have done and will continue to do in my life. I offer You sacrifices of thanksgiving and sing joyfully about Your glorious acts.

Father, before I even pray about my healing, You have already answered my prayers, for Your word states that before I call, You will answer; and yet while I am still speaking, You will hear. I thank You, Father, for this kind of relationship that You and I have, that You are mindful of me. Father, You are the All-Knowing Physician Jehovah Rapha (The Lord Who Heals) who can heal and deliver me from any disease. I bring before You this tinnitus in my ears, vertigo, dizziness, and problems with my balance due to this ear disease. At times, I feel like the room is spinning, and I cannot control that feeling, but what I *can* control is calling on the name of Jesus every time it occurs. There is power in the name of Jesus!

Father, stop my immune system from attacking itself and causing damage to my body tissues. Touch my immune cells and allow them to protect me from germ cells that invade my body and cause it to become a virus or bacteria that leads to inner ear disease. Father, smother and release the inflammation in my blood vessels, repair my inner ear tissue damage, and stop the hearing loss. Father, I ask that You slow down the progression of this disease so that I will not have to wear a hearing aid or have cochlear implants.

I trust in You, and I know that You are with me at all times. I thank You for never leaving me nor forsaking me, Father. I decree and declare my nervous and immune systems, along with sensory hair, blood, and immune cells, will be in harmony with the design You established for their functionality.

According to Your Word, Jesus was wounded for my transgressions, He was bruised for my iniquities, and the chastisement of my peace was upon Him, and by His stripes, **I AM HEALED!** Death and life are in the power of the tongue, so I speak life over my body. I decree and declare prosperity of healing over my body. In Jesus' name.

Whatever medication(s) or hearing devices I am prescribed, I pray that I will not have any side effects, and it will help me, not further harm me, in the name of Jesus. I pray that You give the otolaryngologist, audiologist, and/or rheumatologist that I am a patient of, or will be a patient of, wisdom, knowledge, and understanding of the best treatment for me. I thank You in advance for my complete healing and for being The God Who Is There (Jehovah-Shammah). Amen!

{Psalm 99:9, Psalm 107:21-22, Isaiah 65:24, Psalm 8:4, Romans 11:33, Matthew 9:12, Exodus 15:26, Proverbs 3:5, Hebrew 13:5, Job 22:28, Isaiah 53:5, Proverbs 18:21, 3 John 2, Ezekiel 45:38} NKJV

BALO'S DISEASE

I praise You, Lord, for Your great love and for the wonderful things You have done for me. From the rising of the sun to its going down, Your name is to be praised, Lord. I praise You with my whole heart and soul, God. I bless You, God, every chance I get. My lungs expand with Your praise.

Father, I am so grateful for Your proximity to me when I am hurting. I come humbly before You, requesting that You touch and mend every aspect of my body that needs it. I ask that You calm my muscles so they will stop spasming. Relieve me from the painful headaches and fevers I experience.

Increase mobility in parts of my body that are weak. Strengthen my brain so that I will not have difficulty processing information with my memory and language skills. I pray that whatever damage this disorder caused to my central nervous system will not progress. Father, cancel every assignment that Satan has over my body and life.

As a child of the Most-High God, You have given me the keys (authority) of the kingdom of heaven; and whatever I bind (forbid, declare to be improper and unlawful) on earth will have (already) been bound in heaven, and whatever you loose (permit, declare lawful) on earth will have (already) been loosed in heaven. I bind this rare and progressive disorder, and I loose total healing, strength, deliverance, and restoration in my body. I decree and declare my central nervous and muscular systems, along with my oligodendrocytes (uh-li-gow-den-druh-sites) cells, will be in harmony with the design You established for their functionality.

According to Your Word, Jesus was wounded for my transgressions, He was bruised for my iniquities, and the chastisement of my peace was upon Him, and by His stripes, **I AM HEALED!** Death and life are in the power of the tongue, so I speak life over my body. I decree and declare prosperity of healing over my body. In Jesus' name.

Whatever medication(s) I am prescribed, I pray that I will not have any side effects and it will help me, not further harm me, in the name of Jesus. I thank You, Father, for Your never-ending love and care for me. I am a warrior, and I will overcome this affliction with You by my side every step of the way. For many are the afflictions of the righteous, but You, Lord, will deliver me out of them all. You are My Strength and My Song, and I love You, Father God. Amen!

{Psalm 107:21, Psalm 113:3, Psalm 111:1, Romans 1:12 (AMP), Psalm 34:1 (MSG), Matthew 16:19, Job 22:28, Isaiah 53:5, Proverbs 18:21, 3 John 2, Proverbs 34:19, Isaiah 12:2} NKJV

BECHET'S DISEASE

Before I ask for anything, Father, I come before You, giving You praise and honor. Lord, I praise You, for You are good. I sing praises to Your name, for it is pleasant. Great are You, Lord, and greatly to be praised, and Your greatness is unsearchable. I praise You, for I am fearfully and wonderfully made; marvelous are Your works, and that my soul knows very well. I know that Your Word states that anxiety in the heart of man causes depression, but a good word makes it glad.

Father, I'm calling upon You because I feel like my joy is being robbed because of this rare disorder. I want to have a merry heart because it does good like medicine, and to have a broken spirit does not. It just dries up the bones and makes me weak. Father, turn my discomfort into comfort so that I can live a long and healthy life. I ask that You smother and release the inflammation of my blood vessels so they will stop restricting my blood flow and causing damage to my vital organs and tissues. Alleviate and eliminate the painful sores in my genitals, mouth, joints, and skin. Heal my digestive system so that the diarrhea, bleeding, and abdominal pain can stop. Protect my brain from being attacked by this disorder so that I won't experience fevers, poor balance, headaches, disorientation, or a stroke. Lord, You are good, a stronghold in the day of trouble, and You know those who trust in You.

I put my total trust in You, Lord, for healing and restoration. I decree and declare that my circulatory, digestive, integumentary, central nervous, and lymphatic systems, along with my blood and immune systems, will be in harmony with the design You established for their functionality.

According to Your Word, Jesus was wounded for my transgressions, He was bruised for my iniquities, and the chastisement of my peace was upon Him, and by His stripes, **I AM HEALED!** Death and life are in the power of the tongue, so I speak life over my body. I decree and declare prosperity of healing over my body. In Jesus' name.

Whatever medication(s) I am prescribed, I pray that I will not have any side effects and it will help me, not further harm me, in the name

of Jesus. Heal me, O Lord, and I shall be healed. I thank You in advance that this disorder and the symptoms have been uprooted from my body, and healing is taking place right now as I speak. Thank You for being Omnipotent (All-Knowing) and Omniscient (All-Powerful), God. Amen!

{Psalm 135:3, Psalm 145:3, Psalm 139:14, Proverbs 12:25, Proverbs 17:22, Nahum 1:7, Jeremiah 17:14, Job 22:28, Isaiah 53:5, Proverbs 18:21, 3 John 2, Romans 11:33, Jeremiah 32:17} NKJV

BULLOUS PEMPHIGOID

I will exalt You, my God, O King, and (with gratitude and submissive wonder) I will bless Your name forever and ever. Every day I will bless You and lovingly praise You; yes (with awe-inspired reverence) I will praise Your name forever and forever. I will praise You, Lord! For it is good to sing praises to my God; for it is pleasant and praise is beautiful. I love You, Father, with all my heart, with all my soul, with all my strength, and with my mind.

I believe that all things are possible to those who believe. For with You, God, nothing is ever impossible. No word from God shall be without power or impossible of fulfillment. I come boldly to the throne of grace that I may obtain mercy and grace for help in my time of need. This disorder has caused my immune system to attack my healthy cells in my skin and mouth, and now I have blisters and sores.

Decrease and resolve the widespread blisters on my legs, groin, arms, abdomen, armpits, back, chest, legs, and/or in my mouth. Father, I am asking that You decrease and relieve me from the mild to intense itching and rash on my skin. Statistics say that this skin disorder goes away on its own in a few months, but it can take years for it to clear up. Father, I pray that my condition will not last for years and that when I go into remission, I will stay in remission and not have to continue treatment as others do.

Stretch forth Your healing hands, Father, so that the blisters will not rupture and become infected and cause me to have sepsis. I decree and declare that my integumentary system, along with my blood and immune system cells, will be in harmony with the design You established for their functionality.

According to Your Word, Jesus was wounded for my transgressions, He was bruised for my iniquities, and the chastisement of my peace was upon Him, and by His stripes, **I AM HEALED!** Death and life are in the power of the tongue, so I speak life over my body. I decree and declare prosperity of healing over my body. In Jesus' name.

Whatever medication(s) I am prescribed, I pray that I will not have any side effects and it will help me, not further harm me, in the name of Jesus. Thank You, Father, for allowing me to cast all my cares upon You, for You care for me.

Lord, You are my rock, my fortress, and my deliverer, my God, my strength in whom I will trust. Amen!

{Psalm 145:1-2, Psalm 147:1, Luke 10:27, Luke 1:37, Hebrews 4:16, Job 22:28, Isaiah 53:5, Proverbs 18:21, 3 John 2, 1 Peter 5:7, Psalms 18:2} NKJV

CELIAC DISEASE

I praise Your name, Lord, for Your name is exalted; Your glory is above the earth and heaven. You are the Alpha and the Omega, the Beginning, and the End, the First and the Last. I thank You, Father, that You are before all things, and in You all things exist. Ah, Lord God! Behold, You have made the heavens and the earth by Your great power and outstretched arm. There is nothing too hard for You.

I am asking for relief from the symptoms of diarrhea, abdominal pain, bloating/gas, nausea, vomiting, and constipation that I or my child is experiencing. Boost our energy so we will be alert during times when we are fatigued. Please clear up and take away the itchy/blistery skin rash and mouth sores we have. Decrease and eliminate the joint pain and headaches so we can function well. Father, increase our iriaeficiency and decrease our elevated liver enzymes.

Strengthen, heal, and deliver me and my child from this disease.

Your word tells me that whatever things I ask in prayer and believing, I will receive. Heal me, O Lord, and I shall be healed. I decree and declare that my digestive, skeletal, and integumentary systems, along with blood and immune system cells, will be in harmony with the design You established for their functionality.

According to Your Word, Jesus was wounded for my transgressions, He was bruised for my iniquities, and the chastisement of my peace was upon Him, and by His stripes, **I AM HEALED!** Death and life are in the power of the tongue, so I speak life over my body. I decree and declare prosperity of healing over my body. In Jesus' name.

Whatever medication(s) I am prescribed, I pray that I will not have any side effects and it will help me, not further harm me, in the name of Jesus. I pray that You help me make the right choices concerning the food that I eat so that I will not cause the symptoms to return. You, Lord, are my strength and my shield; my heart trusts in You, and I am helped; therefore, my heart greatly rejoices, and with my song, I will praise You. Blessed be the Lord because You have heard the voice of my supplications. Thank You for being a Wonderful and Mighty God. Amen!

{Psalm 148:13 {KJV}, Revelation 22:13, Colossians 1:17, Jeremiah 32:17, Matthew 21:22, Jeremiah 17:14, Job 22:28, Isaiah 53:5, Proverbs 18:21, 3 John 2, Psalm 28:7, Psalm 23:3, Psalm 28:6, Isaiah 9:6} NKJV

CHRONIC INFLAMMATORY DEMYELINATING POLYNEUROPATHY

Lord, You are beautiful beyond description. You are greatly to be praised. You are A to Z. The God who is, the God who was, and the God who is about to arrive. You are sovereign and strong. Father, You are (eternally changeless, always) the same yesterday and today and forever.

I come boldly to Your throne of grace, asking for healing from this rare neurological disorder that is causing my nerve roots and peripheral nerves to be inflamed, and causing destruction of the myelin sheath. Father, Your Word states that if I serve You, You will bless my food and water, as well as get rid of my sickness and make sure I live a full and complete life. I put my total faith in You and know that Your word shall not return unto You void, but it shall accomplish what You please. Father, I pray that You decrease and eliminate the pain, burning, tingling, and numbness that I am having due to this disease.

Touch my vision so that I can see clearly and not double. Enhance the connection between my body and brain, so that I can regain my reflexes. Strengthen the weakened muscles in my legs so that I won't continue to be clumsy and have difficulty walking. Give me strength like never before, Father, as I battle with this fatigue.

I thank You for giving me the keys (authority) of the kingdom of heaven; and whatever I bind (forbid, declare to be improper and unlawful) on earth will (already) be bound in heaven, and whatever I loose (permit, declare lawful) on earth will have (already) been loosed in heaven. I decree and declare that my central nervous and muscular systems, along with my blood and immune system cells, will be in harmony with the design You established for their functionality.

According to Your Word, Jesus was wounded for my transgressions, He was bruised for my iniquities, and the chastisement of my peace was upon Him, and by His stripes, **I AM HEALED!** Death and life are in the power of the tongue, so I speak life over my situation. I decree and declare prosperity of healing over my body. In Jesus' name.

Whatever medication(s) I am prescribed, I pray that I will not have any side effects and it will help me, not further harm me, in the name of Jesus. Thank You for being a Faithful and Merciful God. Amen!

{Psalm 96:4 (TLB), Revelation 1:8 (MSG), Hebrews 4:16, Exodus 23:25 (MSG), Isaiah 55:11, Matthew 16:19, Job 22:28, Isaiah 53:5, Proverbs 18:21, 3 John 2, Deuteronomy 7:9, Psalm 116:5} NKJV

COGAN'S SYNDROME

Father, You are a Faithful God who keeps covenant and mercy for a thousand generations with those who love You and keep Your commandments. You are the true God, an everlasting king, and there is no one higher than You. O Lord, God of my salvation, I have cried out day and night before You concerning this disease. Father, You are the All-Knowing Physician, Jehovah Rapha (The Lord Who Heals), who is able to heal and deliver me from this rare autoimmune disease.

Jesus went to Galilee, teaching the gospel and healing every sickness and disease–among the people. If He did it for them, I trust and believe He can do it for me. I'm asking in faith, Father, that You stop the narrowing of my blood vessels, so that my blood can flow without restrictions and cause no further damage to my tissues and vital organs. Smother and release the inflammation in my eyes, ears, blood vessels, joints, and muscles. Decrease and eliminate the pain in my ears, eyes, joints, and muscles, along with the headaches, Father.

I ask that You increase my vision and decrease the excess tear production. Relieve the pressure in my ears and help me to find something that will distract my brain, so that I can reduce the tinnitus that I am having. Please stretch forth Your healing hands so that if I have hearing loss, it will be temporary and not permanent, Father. Stop the vertigo and dizziness, so it will not contribute to me losing my balance.

Protect my heart so that I won't develop any heart problems due to this rare autoimmune disease. I know that this disease causes periods of relapse. Father, touch my body so that I will not have any relapses but go into remission and stay in remission until You deliver me completely from this disease. I decree and declare that my nervous, circulatory, and musculoskeletal systems, along with endothelial (endow-thee-lee-uhl), blood, and immune system cells, will be in harmony with the design You established for their functionality.

According to Your Word, Jesus was wounded for my transgressions, He was bruised for my iniquities, and the chastisement of my peace was upon Him, and by His stripes, **I AM HEALED!**

Death and life are in the power of the tongue, so I speak life over my body. I decree and declare prosperity of healing over my body. In Jesus' name.

Whatever medication(s) I am prescribed, I pray that I will not have any side effects and it will help me, not further harm me, in the name of Jesus. I thank You, Father, that I am more valuable to You than the birds in the air. All things are possible with You, Father, so I put all my faith in You that my healing will spring forth speedily. Your word shall not return unto You void, but it shall accomplish what You please. Thank You for being a Good Shepherd and my Restorer Father. Amen!

{Deuteronomy 7:9, Jeremiah 10:10, Psalm 88:1, Romans 11:33, Matthew 9:12, Exodus 15:26, Matthew 4:23, James 1:6, Job 22:28, Isaiah 53:5, Proverbs 18:21, 3 John 2, Matthew 6:26, Mark 9:23, Isaiah 58:8a, Isaiah 55:11, John 10:11, Psalm 23:3} NKJV

CREST SYNDROME

You are worthy, O Lord, to receive glory and honor and power, for You created all things, and by Your will, they exist and were created. You are The God Who Is, The God Who Was, and The God Who Is About To Arrive. You are the sovereign, strong God. Father, Your healing powers are unparalleled. I ask that Your divine touch rest upon my body as I am battling with this systemic connective tissue disease.

I know that I am a child of the Most High God. You have given me the authority and power to trample upon servants and scorpions and over all the power of the enemy, and nothing shall in any way harm me. I am calling on You, Father, asking that You heal, rejuvenate, and restore my body from this disease. Smother and release the inflammation in my skin and joints. Decrease the amount of infection and ulcers on my fingertips and toes, and eliminate the pain that comes along with it. Stop the dyspnea and allow my breathing to return to normal.

It is difficult and painful to swallow because of this disease, so please allow the foods and liquids to go down smoothly and easier because I don't want to continue to have esophageal discomfort. Relieve me from the discomfort of diarrhea, nausea, constipation, and abdominal pain, Father. Limit the amount of spasm attacks of my blood vessels when my hands and feet get cold. Help me to stay calm and stress-free, as much as possible, so that I will not cause my blood vessels to spasm.

This disease has caused me to have deformed hands. When people start to stare, I ask that You help me to stay calm and not say anything that is not like You. At that time, if it is Your will, allow me the opportunity to tell them about the disease and to share my testimony about how good You are.

Father, slow down the progression of this disease so that I will not have any further damage to my kidneys, lungs, and/or heart. Limit the amount of flare-ups and prevent the wasting away of the underlying soft tissue. I decree and declare that my cardiovascular, digestive, integumentary, skeletal, respiratory, and urinary systems, along with my blood and immune system cells, will be in harmony with the design You established for their functionality.

According to Your Word, Jesus was wounded for my transgressions, He was bruised for my iniquities, and the chastisement of my peace was upon Him, and by His stripes, **I AM HEALED!** Death and life are in the power of the tongue, so I speak life over my situation. I decree and declare prosperity of healing over my body. In Jesus' name.

Whatever medication(s) I am prescribed, I pray that I will not have any side effects and it will help me, not further harm me, in the name of Jesus. I thank You, Father, for delivering me from all my afflictions.

No matter how my hands, face, or skin look, I praise You for making me so wonderfully complex. Your workmanship is marvelous. I will continue to trust in You and lean on You for comfort and support. You are a good Father, my Rock, and my Strength. Amen!

{Revelation 4:11, Revelation 1:8 (MSG), John 1:12 (AMP), Luke 10:19 (AMP), Isaiah 53:5, Proverbs 18:21, 3 John 2, Job 22:28, Psalm 34:19, Psalm 139:14 (AMP), Proverbs 3:5, 2 Corinthians 1:3-4, Proverbs 31:3, Isaiah 12:2, Psalm 46:1} NKJV

CROHN'S DISEASE

Holy, holy, holy are You, Lord, the Almighty (the Omnipotent, the Ruler of all) who was and who is to come {the Unchanging, Eternal God}. Great and wonderful and awe-inspiring are Your works, O Lord God, the Almighty (the Omnipotent, the Ruler of all); righteous and true are Your ways, O King of the nations! Who is like You among the gods, O Lord, glorious in holiness, awesome in splendor, performing great wonders?

Father, I have been battling with this chronic inflammatory bowel disease, and it is very overwhelming and stressful to deal with. This disease is causing me to have persistent diarrhea, blood in my stools, and/or rectal bleeding. At other times, I am experiencing constipation, an urgent need to move my bowels, and/or incomplete bowel evacuation. Father, I ask that You decrease and eliminate the pain in my abdomen and joints that I am experiencing. Smother and release the inflammation in my gastrointestinal tract, eyes, liver, joints, skin, and bile ducts.

Take away the fevers, mouth sores, and skin rashes/sores that I am suffering from. Touch my body so that it can produce normal amounts of healthy red blood cells, to get enough oxygen-rich blood, so that I won't continue to be anemic. Increase my appetite and stop me from losing unwanted weight. If I have to change my diet so that I won't have any flare-ups, I ask that You help me to be diligent and persistent with the diet.

Give me strength and energy when I am feeling lethargic and fatigued. Father, because of this disease, my overall health and quality of life are being affected. I am seeking help from You, Father, with this non-curable disease.

I thank You that I can lift my eyes to the hills from where my help comes. My help comes from You, Lord, who made the heaven and earth. My desire is to be completely healed from the crown of my head to the soles of my feet. Your Word says that when I decree a thing, it shall be established unto me. So, I decree and declare that my digestive, muscular, urinary, integumentary, and reproductive systems, along with my blood and immune system cells,

will be in harmony with the design You established for their functionality.

According to Your Word, Jesus was wounded for my transgressions, He was bruised for my iniquities, and the chastisement of my peace was upon Him, and by His stripes, **I AM HEALED!** Death and life are in the power of the tongue, so I speak life over my body. I decree and declare prosperity of healing over my body. In Jesus' name.

Whatever medication(s) I am prescribed, I pray that I will not have any side effects and it will help me, not further harm me, in the name of Jesus. Now that I have cast my cares upon You, Father, I thank You in advance for hearing and answering my prayer. I am grateful to You, Lord, for my life, even when I am faced with difficulties. I thank You for being the Giver of Life and my Anchor. Amen!

{Revelation 4:8 (AMP), Revelation 15:3 (AMP), Exodus 15:11, Psalm 121:1-2,

Job 22:28, Isaiah 53:5, Proverbs 18:21, 3 John 2, 1 Peter 5:7, Job 33:4, Hebrews 6:19} NKJV

DERMATOMYOSITIS

Blessed be my Rock! Be exalted, God, The Rock of my Salvation! I sing to You, Lord, for You are great and greatly to be praised. Father, You are Infallible. Honor and majesty are before You, Lord, and glory is due to You.

I give thanks to You, Lord, for You are good, and Your mercy endures forever. Father, according to Your Word, whatever things I ask in prayer, believing, I will receive. I am asking in faith that You smother and release the inflammation in my blood vessels under my skin and in my muscles. Strengthen the weakened muscles in my shoulders, hips, back, and neck. Clear up the rash on my cheeks, back, eyelids, nose, knees, upper chest, knuckles, and/or elbows.

Father, I am having difficulty swallowing, so I ask that You strengthen my throat muscles and allow swallowing to be easy for me. I am having difficulties rising from a seated position, Father, so allow me to rise easily from a seated position. When I am fatigued, give me the energy and strength to go about my day and perform my daily activities.

Decrease and eliminate the pain in my muscles, Father. I cancel every assignment of sickness and disease that Satan is trying to attack my body with. I thank You, Father, that I am a child of Yours, and Your desire is for me to be healed. I decree and declare that my integumentary, muscular, and digestive systems, along with my blood and immune system cells, will be in harmony with the design You established for their functionality.

According to Your Word, Jesus was wounded for my transgressions, He was bruised for my iniquities, and the chastisement of my peace was upon Him, and by His stripes, **I AM HEALED!** Death and life are in the power of the tongue, so I speak life over my body. I decree and declare prosperity of healing over my body. In Jesus' name.

Whatever medication(s) I am prescribed, I pray that I will not have any side effects and it will help me, not further harm me, in the name of Jesus. I thank You that my healing shall spring forth speedily. Thank You for never leaving me nor forsaking me, for You are the Lord Who Is There.

{2 Samuel 22:47, Psalm 145:3, Isaiah 43:15, I Chronicles 16:27-34, Matthew 21:22, John 1:12 (AMP), Job 22:28, Isaiah 53:5, Proverbs 18:21, 3 John 2, Isaiah 58:8a, Deuteronomy 31:6, Ezekiel 48:35} NKJV

DISCOID LUPUS

Blessed are You, Lord God of Israel, our Father, forever and ever. Yours, O Lord, is the greatness, the power and the glory, the victory, and the majesty; for all that is in heaven and in earth is Yours; Yours is the kingdom, O Lord, and You are exalted as head over all. Both riches and honor come from You, and You reign over all. In Your hand is power and might. In Your hand, it is to make great and to give strength to all.

Now, therefore, my God, I thank You and praise Your glorious name. Thank You that I am wonderfully made; marvelous are Your works, and that my soul knows very well. Father, I am casting all my cares [all my anxieties, all my worries, and all my concerns], once and for all, on You, for You care about me [with deepest affection] and watch over me very carefully.

Father, my immune system is attacking itself and causing me to have scaling and crusty patches that are inflamed, peeling of the skin, thinning of the skin, skin pigmentation, thickening of the scalp, and hair loss.

Stop my immune system from attacking my healthy skin so that it can prevent further inflammation on my skin and scalp. Father, this disease is known for scarring, so I ask that You protect my skin and scalp from forming scars. It can be a bit uncomfortable when people are staring at me and thinking I'm contagious because they can see the scars and discoloration on my skin. When they are staring, and if it is Your will, allow me the opportunity to share with them what the disease is and how You are there for me.

I thank You for making me so wonderfully complex! Your workmanship is marvelous. Father, it has been documented that anyone who's battling with discoid lupus faces an increased risk of developing skin cancer. Heal and deliver me from discoid lupus so that I won't be one of the ones who have a cancer diagnosis.

Help me do my part by protecting my skin from the beautiful sun that You made by wearing sunscreen when needed. I decree and declare that my integumentary and immune systems, along with my blood and immune system cells, will be in harmony with the design You established for their functionality.

According to Your Word, Jesus was wounded for my transgressions, He was bruised for my iniquities, and the chastisement of my peace was upon Him, and by His stripes, **I AM HEALED!** Death and life are in the power of the tongue, so I speak life over my

body. I decree and declare prosperity of healing over my body. In Jesus' name.

Whatever medication(s) I am prescribed, I pray that I will not have any side effects and that it will help me, not further harm me, in the name of Jesus. I cancel every assignment and destruction that Satan has over my body, and I denounce it in the name of Jesus. I will walk in good health, and I am rejuvenated because You are the All-Knowing Physician and the source of all healing. Amen!

{1 Chronicles 29:10-13, Psalm 139:14 (AMP), 1 Peter 5:7, Psalm 139:14 9(NLT), Isaiah 53:5, Proverbs 18:21, 3 John 2, Romans 11:33, Matthew 9:12} NKJV

ENDOMETRIOSIS

I will stand up and bless You, God, forever and ever! Blessed be Your glorious name, which is exalted above all blessing and praise! You alone are the Lord; You have made heaven, the heavens, with all their host, the earth and everything on it, the seas and all that is in them, and You preserve them all. The host of heaven worships You.

The Spirit of God has made me, and the breath of the Almighty gives me life. Keep me as the apple of Your eye, Father. I come boldly to the throne of grace that I may obtain mercy and find grace to help in time of need. I am experiencing unbearable pain before, during, and after my menses from this menstrual disease.

There are days when it is painful to walk, and all I want to do is lie in bed and cry, wishing this were over, with no menstrual cycle again in life. I ask that You release the pressure on my nerves so that I won't have constant throbbing, sharp, and/or stabbing pain walking and doing daily activities. It is very difficult to go to school and/or work when feeling like this because all I am focusing on is the pain and the task at hand, Father. The discomfort that I am experiencing feels like something is pulling on the organs in my pelvic region, and it is very uncomfortable and severely painful.

The over-the-counter pain medications are not working anymore. Father, stretch forth Your healing hands to deliver, strengthen, and restore my body. I ask that You decrease and eliminate the pain during, before, and/or after my menses; and during or after intercourse with my spouse. Relieve me from abdominal pain, body aches, and headaches, along with pain associated with my lower back, legs, pelvis, urination, bowel movements, and hip pain that radiates to my buttocks. Smother and release the inflammation within my pelvic cavity so that it will not increase the risk of causing damage to my nerves and developing neuropathy. Stop the overproduction of estrogen in my body so that I won't continue to gain weight.

Bring to a minimum and stop the gastrointestinal distress that I am having due to this disease. Father, I do not want to suffer from infertility and would like to have a child or children. Touch my body and remove anything that will cause me to not have a regular ovulation. Allow my body to be able to conceive and be fruitful and multiply and sustain my pregnancy. Give me the energy and strength from the fatigue that I have, so that I can be alert and perform my daily activities.

I know that nothing is impossible with You, Father, so I ask that You protect my bladder, appendix, intestines, lungs, brain, kidneys, and diaphragm from being attacked by this awful disease. I decree and declare that my reproductive, digestive, urinary, and musculoskeletal systems, along with my endometrial cells, blood, and immune system cells, will be in harmony with the design You established for their functionality.

According to Your Word, Jesus was wounded for my transgressions, He was bruised for my iniquities, and the chastisement of my peace was upon Him, and by His stripes, **I AM HEALED!** Death and life are in the power of the tongue, so I speak life over my body. I decree and declare prosperity of healing over my body. In Jesus' name.

Whatever medication(s) I am prescribed, I pray that I will not have any side effects and it will help me, not further harm me, in the name of Jesus. When the righteous cry (for help), You hear and rescue them from all their distress and troubles. I thank You, Father, for nursing me back to health when I am at my worst and for soothing my pains and worries from this disease. Thank You for renewing strength in my body when I am weak and for regenerating my cells. I thank You in advance for hearing my prayers and seeing my tears, for surely You will heal me, Father. For You are the All-Knowing Physician (Jehovah Rapha), The One Who Heals. Amen!

{Nehemiah 9:5-6, Job 33:4, Psalm 17:8, Hebrews 4:16, Genesis 9:7, Luke 1:37, Job 22:28, Isaiah 53:5, 3 John 2, Psalm 34:17 (AMP), Psalm 41:3, Isaiah 40:29, 2 Kings 20:5, Romans 11:33, Matthew 9:12, Exodus 15:26} NKJV

ESSENTIAL MIXED CRYOGLOBULINEMIA

I will praise You, Lord, according to Your righteousness, and will sing praise to the name of the Lord Most High. I will praise You, O Lord, with my whole heart; I will tell of all Your marvelous works. I will be glad and rejoice in You, and I will sing praise to Your name, O Most High. I lift up my eyes to the hills from whence comes my help. My help comes from the Lord, who made heaven and earth.

Giver of Life, I ask that You touch my body and cause my abnormal antibodies to become normal again so they will not clump together and become solid or gel-like. Father, please prevent the proteins from clumping together in my bloodstream, as it is preventing blood flow to my muscles, organs, and joints. Allow my blood to flow freely in my body. Smother the inflammation in my blood vessels that have been affected by this disorder and prevent any further damage to my surrounding tissue. Decrease and eliminate the pain in my joints, muscles, and abdomen.

Stop the bleeding from underneath my skin and heal the skin lesions, Father. Heal and restore my body from the other conditions related to this disorder. I decree that my cardiovascular, musculoskeletal, urinary, lymphatic, nervous, integumentary, digestive, and respiratory systems, along with my blood and immune system cells, will be in harmony with the design You established for their functionality.

According to Your Word, Jesus was wounded for my

transgressions, He was bruised for my iniquities, and the chastisement of my peace was upon Him, and by His stripes, **I AM HEALED!** Death and life are in the power of the tongue, so I speak life over my body. I decree and declare prosperity of healing over my body. In Jesus' name.

Whatever medication(s) I am prescribed, I pray that I will not have any side effects and it will help me, not further harm me, in the name of Jesus. I thank You in advance that my healing shall spring forth speedily, Everlasting Father. Amen!

{Psalm 7:17, Psalm 9:1-2, Psalm 121:1-2, Job 33:4, Isaiah 26:4, Job 22:28, Isaiah 53:5, Proverbs 18:21, 3 John 2, Isaiah 58:8a, Isaiah 9:6} NKJV

GRANULOMATOSIS WITH POLYANGIITIS (ALSO WEGENER'S GRANULOMATOSIS)

You, Lord, are my rock and my fortress and my deliverer; my God, my strength, in whom I will trust; my shield and the horn of my salvation, my stronghold. I sing praises to You, Lord, and give thanks in the remembrance of Your holy name. Blessed be the Lord because You have heard the voice of my supplications. I thank You, Lord, that You are the God who bears my burdens day by day.

You know what I am dealing with and how I am feeling on a daily basis, for You are the All-Knowing God. Father, I come to You asking that You smother and release the inflammation of my blood vessels so that I won't continue to experience issues with my lungs, kidneys, and sinuses. Cause my blood to flow freely and unrestricted so that it won't damage any of my vital organs and tissues. Relieve my body from the symptoms of fatigue, night sweats, fevers, joint pain, loss of appetite, skin sores, and eye problems, Father.

My heart's desire is to be in remission and not to have relapses. Father, I ask that You turn my discomfort to comfort and heal me from this chronic disorder. I decree and declare that my cardiovascular, integumentary, respiratory, urinary, and musculoskeletal systems, along with my blood and immune system cells, will be in harmony with the design You established for their functionality.

According to Your Word, Jesus was wounded for my transgressions, He was bruised for my iniquities, and the chastisement of my peace was upon Him, and by His stripes, **I AM HEALED!** Death and life are in the power of the tongue, so I speak life over my body. I decree and declare prosperity of healing over my body. In Jesus' name.

Whatever medication(s) I am prescribed, I pray that I will not have any side effects and it will help me, not further harm me, in the name of Jesus. I believe and trust in You, Lord, that You will restore my health and heal me. I thank You, Father, that Your Word will not return unto You void but shall accomplish what You please. Blessed be the Lord God, the God of Israel, who only does wonderous things. Amen!

{Psalm 18:2, Psalms 30:4, Psalm 28:6, Psalm 68:19 (AMP), Romans 11:33,

Jeremiah 30:17, Exodus 15:26, Job 22:28, Isaiah 53:5, Proverbs 18:21, 3 John 2, Jeremiah 30:17, Isaiah 55:11, Psalm 72:18} NKJV

GRAVES' DISEASE

I will bless You, Lord, at all times; Your praise shall continually be in my mouth. My tongue shall speak of Your righteousness and of Your praise all the day long. Lord, You are my refuge and strength, a very present help in trouble. I lift my eyes to the hills from where my help comes from.

My help comes from You, Lord, who made heaven and earth. Father, You are the All-Knowing Physician Jehovah Rapha (The Lord Who Heals) and can heal and deliver me from any disease. I know that a weapon can be formed against me, but it shall not prosper. I put my trust in You for my healing.

I come before You, Lord, asking You to reduce the amount of thyroid hormones that my body produces so that it will lessen the unpleasant symptoms that I am experiencing. Decrease the abnormal enlarged goiter, so it will go back to the normal size I had before I was diagnosed with Graves' Disease. My muscles are weak due to this disease, so strengthen them so that I won't continue to have difficulty moving my limbs. When I have exophthalmos, please let it return to normal sooner rather than later.

I don't want to have surgery to move my eye back to a normal position and have a portion of the bones surrounding my eye removed. Father, regulate my thyroid hormones so my skin, eyes, muscles, heart, and other organs won't continue to be affected by this disease. Protect my healthy cells from being attacked by my immune system. I decree and declare that my endocrine, muscular, circulatory, nervous, integumentary, reproductive, and immune systems, along with my hormone-secreting cells, blood, and immune system cells, will be in harmony with the design You established for their functionality.

According to Your Word, Jesus was wounded for my transgressions, He was bruised for my iniquities, and the chastisement of my peace was upon Him, and by His stripes, **I AM HEALED!** Death and life are in the power of the tongue, so I speak life over my body. I decree and declare prosperity of healing over my body. In Jesus' name.

Whatever medication(s) I am prescribed, I pray that I will not have any side effects and it will help me, not further harm me, in the name of Jesus. Thank You for being a great, mighty, and awesome God who keeps Your covenant and mercy. Amen!

{Psalm 34:1, Psalm 35:28, Psalm 46:1, Psalm 121:1-2, Exodus 15:26, Psalm 103:3, Isaiah 54:17, Proverbs 3:5, Job 22:28, Isiah 53:5, Proverbs 18:21, 3 John 2, Nehemiah 9:32} NKJV

GUILLAIN-BARRE SYNDROME

For You are great beyond description and greatly to be praised, Lord. Gracious are You, Lord, and righteous. Yes, God, You are merciful. I will exalt You, God, and worship You at Your holy hill, for You, Lord my God, are holy. I find comfort in You, for You are my resting place.

As Your Word states, whatever things I ask in prayer, believing, I will receive. I seek comfort in You, Lord God, who comforts me in all my tribulation. Father, I am seeking You concerning my immune system attacking and causing damage to the myelin of the nerves in my peripheral nervous system. I ask that You heal and restore the myelin so that it will not continue to hinder the communication between my brain and body.

In my time of weakness, Father, You will give me strength because You are my source of strength. I'm asking that You strengthen the weakened muscles in my feet, face, legs, and arms, along with my breathing muscles. When I am fatigued, give me the energy and strength to go about my day and to perform my daily activities. Decrease and eliminate the severe deep muscular pain in my legs and/or back that I am experiencing.

I am also having discomfort in other areas of my body due to this rare neurological disorder. Father, my heart's desire is to be healed and restored from this disorder. I pray that You turn my discomfort into comfort so that I can go back to living a healthy life. I decree and declare that my immune, nervous, muscular, digestive, and respiratory systems, along with my blood and immune system cells, will be in harmony with the design You established for their functionality.

According to Your Word, Jesus was wounded for my transgressions, He was bruised for my iniquities, and the chastisement of my peace was upon Him, and by His stripes, **I AM HEALED!** Death and life are in the power of the tongue, so I speak life over my body. I decree and declare prosperity of healing over my body. In Jesus' name.

Whatever medication(s) I am prescribed, I pray that I will not have any side effects and it will help me, not further harm me, in the name of Jesus. I trust and believe that You will send Your Word to heal and deliver me from this disorder, Father. I thank You that You are the God who heals all diseases. Amen!

{Psalm 96:4 (TLB), Psalm 116:5, Psalm 99:9, Matthew 21:22, 2 Corinthians 1:4, 2 Corinthians 12:9, Job 22:28, Isaiah 53:5, Proverbs 18:21, 3 John 2, Psalm 107:20, Psalm 103:3} NKJV

HASHIMOTO'S THYROIDITIS

I will sing to the Lord as long as I live; I will sing praises to You, God, while I have my being. I give You thanks, Lord, for You are good! For Your mercy endures forever. I thank You, Lord, for being my Creator. God, You alone are wise, be glory through Jesus Christ forever.

Father, Your Word says, "Come to me, all who labor and are heavy laden, and I will give you rest." As I cast my cares upon You, I am seeking Your promised rest, Father. When I cry out to You for help, You hear me and will rescue me from my distress and troubles. Father, touch my immune system so that it can protect and not attack and destroy my thyroid gland.

Stop my body from developing antibodies that cause damage to my thyroid gland. Smother and release the inflammation in my thyroid gland, so that it will not continue to get bigger and cause me to have pressure, neck discomfort, or trouble swallowing. Allow my thyroid gland to make enough thyroid hormones so that it won't continue to cause further damage. I am asking for strength and healing in my ailing body.

This disorder is causing a lot of unwanted symptoms in my body. This disorder has me fatigued on a daily basis, so give me strength and energy to perform my daily activities. Loosen my bowels, so that I will no longer be constipated. Decrease and eliminate the aches and pain in my muscles and joints.

Stop my weight from fluctuating and help me to be consistent with my lifestyle changes in dieting and exercising. Stop the follicles in my scalp from being damaged and causing thinning or loss of hair. Strengthen and stimulate the follicles so that they can stay healthy, and new hair can start to grow back. I exercise my authority over the enemy, and nothing will (in any way) harm me.

With Your help, I can conquer this disorder because I am more than a conqueror. Father, I know that You have great plans for my life, plans to take care of me, not abandon me, and plans to give me the future I hope for. For the Word of God is living, active, and full of power (making it operative, energizing, and effective). I decree and declare that my endocrine, musculoskeletal, nervous, integumentary, and digestive systems, along with hormone-secreting, blood, and immune system cells, will be in harmony with the design You established for their functionality.

According to Your Word, Jesus was wounded for my transgressions, He was bruised for my iniquities, and the chastisement of my peace was upon Him, and by His stripes, **I AM HEALED!** Death and life are in the power of the tongue, so I speak life over my body. I decree and declare prosperity of healing over my body. In Jesus' name.

Whatever medication(s) I am prescribed, I pray that I will not have any side effects and it will help me, not further harm me, in the name of Jesus. I thank You for being the All-Knowing and All-Powerful God. For You heard my prayer, You have seen my tears; surely You will heal me, Father. Thank You in advance for complete healing and restoration. Amen!

{Psalm 104:33, Psalm 107:1, Isaiah 43:15, Romans 16:27, Matthew 11:28, 1 Peter 5:7, Psalm 34:17, Luke 10:19, Romans 8:37, Jeremiah 29:11 (AMP), Hebrews 4:12 (AMP), Job 22:28, Isaiah 53:5, Proverbs 18:21, 3 John 2, Romans 11:33, Jeremiah 32:17, 2 Kings 20:5} NKJV

IGA NEPHROPATHY

I praise You, Lord, for Your great love and for the wonderful things You have done. I offer my sacrifices of thanksgiving, and I sing joyfully about Your glorious acts. I will praise You, Lord, with my whole heart. From the rising of the sun to its going down, Your name is to be praised.

Father, stop the antibodies from building up and settling in my kidneys so that my kidneys can function the way You made them. Smother and release the inflammation in my kidneys, so my kidneys can filter waste from my blood and stop the leaking of blood and protein into my urine. Clear up the foamy urine and make it clear again. Father, decrease and eliminate the pain I'm having in the side of my back beneath my ribs.

Reduce and release the inflammation in my hands and feet. Help me to do whatever I have to do to lower my blood pressure. Give me strength when I am weak and tired, Father. I ask that You stop antibodies from attacking my immune system and causing the pathogens to be invaded. In Jesus' name.

It has been stated that this disease can develop into end-stage kidney failure, and there is no cure. Father, I pray that You will heal and restore my kidneys so that I won't get to the point of end-stage kidney failure and have to be on dialysis or need a kidney transplant.

FOR THOSE ON DIALYSIS

Father, I pray that every time I go to dialysis, you strengthen my body when the process is over. I don't like the way I feel after dialysis. So, I ask in the name of Jesus that You, please take away the risks and side effects of dialysis. For Your Word says that Jesus healed all kinds of sickness and all kinds of diseases among the people. If He did it for them, I believe that He can do it for me as well. So, I decree and declare that my urinary and circulatory systems, along with blood and immune system cells, will be in harmony with the design You established for their functionality.

According to Your Word, Jesus was wounded for my transgressions, He was bruised for my iniquities, and the chastisement of my peace was upon Him, and by His stripes, **I AM HEALED!** Death and life are in the power of the tongue, so I speak life over my body. I decree and declare prosperity of healing over my body. In Jesus' name.

Whatever medication(s) I am prescribed, I pray that I will not get any side effects and it will help me, not further harm me, in the name of Jesus.

I thank You in advance, Father, for taking away this infirmity and healing me completely from the crown of my head to the soles of my feet. Thank You that my prayer will not fall on deaf ears Father, for

You stated that when I cry (for help), You hear and will rescue me from all my distress and troubles. I thank You for being the Good Shepherd. Amen!

{Psalm 107:21-22 (NLT), Psalm 111:1, Psalm 113:3, Job 22:28, Matthew 4:23, Isaiah 53:5, Proverbs 18:21, 3 John 2, Psalm 34:17 (AMP), John 10:11} NKJV

IMMUNE THROMBOCYTOPENIA PURPURA (ITP)

I am making a joyful shout to You, Lord. Serving You with gladness, coming before Your presence with singing. Knowing that You, Lord, are God; it is You who has made me and not myself. I am Your child and the sheep of Your pasture. I enter into Your gates with thanksgiving and into Your courts with praise.

I am thankful to You, and I bless Your name. For You, Lord, are good; Your mercy is everlasting, and Your truth endures to all generations. You are my dwelling place (my refuge, my sanctuary, my stability) in all generations. I trust (confidently) in You, Lord, forever. You are my fortress, my shield, my banner, for You, Lord God, are an everlasting rock (the Rock of Ages).

I come before You, Father, seeking help with this autoimmune bleeding disorder. Stretch forth Your healing hands to strengthen and restore my immune system so that it will not continue to destroy my platelets. Increase the low levels of platelets so my blood can clot and not cause significant bleeding or bruising, Father. Heal, deliver, and restore my body from this bleeding disorder that is causing me to have nosebleeds, bleeding gums, blood in my stool, heavy menses, bruising, and/or petechiae (puh-tee-kee-uh), reddish-purple spots.

I decree and declare that my circulatory, integumentary, and reproductive systems, along with blood and immune system cells, will be in harmony with the design You established for their functionality.

According to Your Word, Jesus was wounded for my transgressions, He was bruised for my iniquities, and the chastisement of my peace was upon Him, and by His stripes, **I AM HEALED!** Death and life are in the power of the tongue, so I speak life over my

situation. I decree and declare prosperity of healing over my body. In Jesus' name.

Whatever medication(s) I am prescribed, I pray that I will not get any side effects and it will help me, not further harm me, in the name of Jesus. I thank You in advance for total and complete healing. I thank You for hearing and answering the effective, fervent prayers, Father. Thank You for being my Healer and my Strength. Amen!

{Psalm 100:1-5, Psalm 90:1 (AMP), Isaiah 26:4 (AMP), Job 22:28, Isaiah 53:5, Proverbs 18:21, 3 John 2, James 5:16b (AMP), Exodus 15:26, Isaiah 12:2} NKJV

INCLUSION BODY MYOSITIS (IBM)

I will praise You, Lord, for You are good; I will sing praises to Your name, for it is pleasant. I will exalt You, my God, O King, and (with gratitude and submissive wonder) I will bless Your name forever and ever. Every day, I will bless You and lovingly praise You. Yes (with awe-inspired reverence), I will praise Your name forever and ever. I come boldly to the throne of grace, that I may obtain mercy and find grace to help in time of need from this muscle disease.

Father, Your Word says, Come to me, all who labor and are heavy laden, and I will give you rest. Thank You, Father, for allowing me to cast all my cares upon You, for You care for me. You are the All-Knowing Physician Jehovah Rapha (The Lord Who Heals) who can heal me from this slow progression disease.

I know that this disease is incurable, Father, but I believe that You can cure me from it. For Your Word tells me that Jesus healed all kinds of sicknesses and diseases among the people. If He did it for them, I believe He can do it for me as well because there is no partiality with Him. Father, decrease and eliminate the pain in my muscles that I am experiencing. Slow down the progression of the muscle atrophy and increase the strength in my muscles, so they won't continue to decline.

Strengthen my weakened muscles so that I can move like I used to without limitations. Smother and release the inflammation in my legs, fingers, wrists, and face. Father, stop my body from attacking its own muscles so that it won't cause any more damage to my muscles. I ask that You give me the strength to endure the physical therapy, exercising, occupational therapy, speech therapy, and fall prevention that I must perform as a source of managing and strengthening the functioning of my muscles.

Take away the difficulty I have swallowing and allow me to swallow with ease. I ask that You pull up and uproot this muscle disease and kill it at the root. I decree and declare that my muscular, nervous, digestive, and respiratory systems, along with my blood and immune system cells, will be in harmony with the design You established for their functionality.

According to Your Word, Jesus was wounded for my transgressions, He was bruised for my iniquities, and the chastisement of my peace was upon Him, and by His stripes, **I AM HEALED!** Death and life are in the power of the tongue, so I speak life over my body. I declare prosperity of healing over my body. In Jesus' name.

Whatever medication(s) I am prescribed, I pray that I will not get any side effects and it will help me, not further harm me, in the name of Jesus. I thank You, Father, for being the Giver of Life and my Anchor. Amen!

{Psalm 135:3, Psalm 145:1-2 (AMP), Hebrews 4:16, Matthew 11:28, 1 Peter 5:7, Romans 11:33, Exodus 15:26, Matthew 4:23, Romans 2:11, Job 22:28, Isaiah 53:5, Proverbs 18:21, 3 John 2, Job 33:4, Hebrews 6:19} NKJV

JUVENILE IDIOPATHIC ARTHRITIS (JIA)

Great is the Lord, and greatly to be praised; Your greatness is unsearchable. Gracious are You, Lord, and righteous; yes, You are merciful. I will bless You, Lord, at all times. Your praise shall continually be in my mouth. Your Word states that when the righteous cry (for help), the Lord hears and rescues them from all their distress and troubles.

I bring my prayers to You concerning **(child's name)**. Father, it's hard seeing **(child's name)** go through this **(name of the arthritis**

your child has), and there is nothing I can do to take it away. I cast all my cares upon You, for You care for me as well as for **(child's name).** So, I'm going to do what I know how to do, and that is pray because the effective, fervent prayers of a righteous man avail much.

(Child's Name) been experiencing pain, swelling, stiffness in joints, fatigue, eye problems, recurring fevers, poor appetite, anemia, and rashes because of this condition. I know that You are the only one who can strengthen, heal, and restore **(child's name)** body and mind. Father, I ask that You smother and release the inflammation in **(child's name)** body. Remove the pain that **(child's name)** is having.

Turn his/her discomfort to comfort and allow **(child's name)** to live a full and healthy life, Father. Your Word states to trust You with all my heart and lean not unto my own understanding. Father, I put **(child's name)** in Your hands.

I decree and declare that **(child's name)'s muscular, respiratory, circulatory, digestive, skeletal, nervous, lymphatic, and integumentary systems, along with (child's name)** blood and immune cells, will be in harmony with the design You established for their functionality.

According to Your Word, Jesus was wounded for **(child's name)** transgressions, He was bruised for **(child's name)** iniquities, and the chastisement of **(child's name)** peace was upon Him, and by His stripes, **MY CHILD IS HEALED!** Death and life are in the power of the tongue, so I speak life over **(child's name)** body. I declare prosperity of healing over **(child's name)** body. In Jesus' name.

Whatever medication(s) **(child's name)** is prescribed, I pray that he/she will not get any side effects and it will help him/her, not further harm him/her, in the name of Jesus. I thank You, Father, that **(child's name)** is blessed and loved by You. I thank You in advance for total and complete healing for **(child's name).** Thank You for being my Burden Bearer. Thank You for answering a mother's prayer for her child in my day of distress. Amen!

{Psalm 145:3, Psalm 116:5, Psalm 34:1, Psalm 34:17 (AMP), 1 Peter 5:7, James 5:16b, Proverbs 3:5, Isaiah 53:5, Proverbs 18:21, 3 John 2, Psalm 68:19 (AMP), Genesis 35:3} NKJV

LAMBERT-EATON MYASTHENIC SYNDROME (LEMS)

I praise You, Lord! For it is good to sing praises to our God; for it is pleasant, and praise is beautiful. As for You, God, Your ways are perfect; Your Word, Lord, is proven; You are a shield to all who trust in You. Ah, Lord God! Behold, You have made the heavens and the earth by Your great power and outstretched arm. There is nothing too hard for You.

I come before You, Father, asking that You touch my neuromuscular junction so that it can stop interfering with the ability of my muscle cells to receive the signals they need from my nerve cells. Allow my nerve cells to release enough chemicals (acetylcholine) and transmit impulses between my nerves and muscles. Strengthen the stiffened and weakened muscles in my arms, shoulders, legs, and hips.

Give me the strength to be able to get out of a chair, walk, run, climb stairs, lift, and push. These are the times when it is hard for me, and I need a touch from Your healing hands. Heal my body from the other symptoms that I am experiencing as well.

(If you have LEMS associated with cancer, add this to your prayer.) Father, I ask that You uproot every cancer cell in my body, and that You kill it at the very root so that it will not metastasize.

I am casting all my cares [all my anxieties, all my worries, and all my concerns], once and for all, on You, for You care about me [with deepest affection] and watch over me very carefully. I decree and declare that my nervous, muscular, digestive, and sensory systems, along with my blood and immune system cells, will be in harmony with the design You established for their functionality. According to Your Word, Jesus was wounded for my transgressions, He was bruised for my iniquities, and the chastisement of my peace was upon Him, and by His stripes, **I AM HEALED!** Death and life are in the power of the tongue, so I speak life over my body. I decree and declare prosperity of healing over my body. In Jesus' name.

Whatever medication(s) I am prescribed, I pray that I will not have any side effects and it will help me, not further harm me, in the name of Jesus. I thank You, Father, for complete healing, renewed strength, and restoration in my body. Now, Lord, what do I wait for? My hope is in You. I thank You for bearing my burden day by day, Lord, for You are my Salvation. Amen!

{Psalm 147:1, Psalm 18:30, Jeremiah 32:17, 1 Peter 5:7 (AMP), Job 22:28, Isaiah 53:5, Proverbs 18:21, 3 John 2, Psalm 39:7, Psalm 68:19 AMP)} NKJV

LUPUS

Your work is honorable and glorious, and Your righteousness endures forever. You have made Your wonderful works to be remembered. You are gracious and full of compassion. You have given food to those who fear You. You will ever be mindful of Your covenant. I will exalt You, Lord, and worship You at Your holy hill, for the Lord my God is holy. I will bless You, Lord, O my soul; and all that is within me, I will bless Your holy name!

Father, I come before You asking that You touch my immune system and stop it from fighting against itself. Stop and repair the damage to my body that this non-curable chronic inflammatory disease has caused. I ask that You protect my immune system from further damage. Heal, strengthen, and restore me. Smother and decrease the inflammation in my glands, joints, muscles, arms, legs, face, and scalp.

Decrease and eliminate any pain in my muscles, joints, chest, and head. When I am worn out and fatigued, give me strength, for Your grace is sufficient for me and Your strength is made perfect in my weakness. Grow back my hair where there was hair loss. Protect my kidneys, heart, and brain from having further damage–that lupus can cause.

I ask that You turn my discomfort to comfort, as I battle with this disease. When I have flares, I ask that they don't last for days or weeks, Father. It has been reported that in remission, lupus activity is not evident, although lupus itself may still be present. So, Father, I ask that if I go into remission, let it be permanent for me.

I thank You in advance for healing me from this awful disease. I decree and declare that my circulatory, digestive, integumentary, nervous, renal, respiratory, and musculoskeletal systems, along with my blood and immune system cells, will be in harmony with the design You established for their functionality.

According to Your Word, Jesus was wounded for my transgressions, He was bruised for my iniquities, and the chastisement of my peace was upon Him, and by His stripes, **I AM HEALED!** Death and life are in the power of the tongue, so I speak life over my body. I decree and declare prosperity of healing over my body. In Jesus' name.

Whatever medication(s) I am prescribed, I pray that I will not have any side effects and it will help me, not further harm me, in the name of Jesus. Father, I will continue earnestly in prayer about my health, being vigilant in it with thanksgiving. I trust in You that You know what is best for me. I believe that Your word shall not return unto You void, but it shall accomplish what You please in the precious and mighty name of Jesus. Thank You for being the Giver of Life and my Anchor. Amen!

{Psalm 111:3-5, Psalm 99:9, Psalm 103:1, Job 22:28, Isaiah 53:5, Proverbs 18:21, 3 John 2, Colossians 4:2, Isaiah 55:11} NKJV

MIXED CONNECTIVE TISSUE DISEASE(MCTD)

You are great beyond description and greatly to be praised, Lord. I worship only You, God. I praise You, Lord! For it is good to sing praises to You, my God; for it is pleasant, and praise is beautiful.

You are worthy, O Lord, to receive glory and honor and power, for You created all things, and by Your will, they exist and were created. I lift up my eyes to the hills from where my help comes from. My help comes from You, Lord, who made the heaven and the earth. Father, You told me to cast all our cares [all our anxieties, all our worries, and all my concerns, once and for all] on You, for You care about me [with deepest affection] and watch over me very carefully.

Your Word states that whatever things I ask in prayer, believing, I will receive. Father, I ask that You stretch forth Your healing hands and heal my body from this overlapping of several connective tissue diseases of systemic lupus erythematosus, scleroderma, polymyositis, and/or rheumatoid arthritis. Smother and release the inflammation throughout my body. Decrease and eliminate the pain in my joints, muscles, hands, fingers, chest, and nerves.

With the malaise and extreme fatigue, it is hard to perform my daily activities, including my job responsibilities. At times, I am mentally tired, agitated, and depressed as a result of this disease. I ask that You help me to have positive thoughts, so that I can calm my emotions. My body is being hit hard due to multiple diseases that have different symptoms.

I ask that You give me strength in my body and give me peace in my mind so that I can live a healthy, productive life. I'm so glad that You are in my life, Father because when I am unstable, You are stable. Father, give me peace; a peace that surpasses all understanding that will guard my heart and mind through Christ Jesus. I look to You, Father because You are the source of all healing.

I decree and declare that my cardiovascular, digestive, integumentary, musculoskeletal, nervous, renal, and respiratory systems, along with my endothelial, epithelial, contractile, neuron, blood, and immune cells, will be in harmony with the design You established for their functionality.

According to Your Word, Jesus was wounded for my transgressions, He was bruised for my iniquities, and the chastisement of my peace was upon Him, and by His stripes, **I AM HEALED!** Death and life are in the power of the tongue, so I speak life over my body. I decree and declare prosperity of healing over my body. In Jesus' name.

Whatever medication(s) I am prescribed, I pray that I will not have any side effects and it will help me, not further harm me, in the name of Jesus. Thank You in advance for healing, strength, and restoration, Father. You are my Strength and my Song. Thank You for being the Prince of Peace. Amen!

{Psalm 96:4 (TLB), Psalm 147:1, Revelation 4:11, Psalm 121:1-2, 1 Peter 5:7 (AMP), 2 Corinthians 12:9, Matthew 21:22,

Philippians 4:7, Job 22:28, Isaiah 53:5, Proverbs 18:21, 3 John 2, Isaiah 12:2, Isaiah 9:6} NKJV

MULTIPLE SCLEROSIS (MS)

O Lord, You are my God. I will exalt You, I will praise Your name, For You have done wonderful things. Your counsels of old are faithfulness and truth. Behold, God, You are my salvation. I will trust and not be afraid, For You, the Lord is my strength and song. You are my Strong Tower. When I run to You, I am safe.

Father, I'm seeking Your face concerning all that I am experiencing with MS and asking for complete healing. I ask that You cure me of this incurable disease so I will not continue to experience these symptoms of cognitive impairments, spasticity, difficulties with balancing, paralysis, bladder problems, migraines, dysesthesia, speech impediments, complete loss of vision, hearing loss and/or depression. Strengthen the weak muscles in my legs, ankles, and feet so that they will not interfere with my walking. When I am fatigued, Father, strengthen and supply my body with energy and give me motivation so that I can perform my daily activities.

Strengthen my brain so that I will not continue to have issues with my memory, learning new things, concentrating, and making any decisions. Father, I ask that You bring back to my remembrance anything that I need to remember that affects my everyday life. I put my trust in You for my comfort, peace, and rest as I battle with these attacks. I decree and declare that my musculoskeletal, nervous, and urinary systems, along with my blood and immune system cells, will be in harmony with the design You established for their functionality.

According to Your Word, Jesus was wounded for my transgressions, He was bruised for my iniquities, and the chastisement of my peace was upon Him, and by His stripes, **I AM HEALED!** Death and life are in the power of the tongue, so I speak life over my body. I decree and declare prosperity of healing over my body. In Jesus' name.

Whatever medication(s) I am prescribed, I pray that I will not have

any side effects and it will help me, not further harm me, in the name of Jesus. When I have to go to physical, occupational, and/or speech therapy, I ask Father that You give me the strength and endurance to perform what is required of me.

I thank You, Father God, in advance for healing, deliverance, strength, and restoration in my body. Thank You for being my Anchor and my Comforter. Amen!

{Isaiah 25:1, Isaiah 12:2, Proverbs 18:10, Job 22:28, Isaiah 53:5, Proverbs 18:21, 3 John 2, Hebrews 6:19, 2 Corinthians 1:3-4} NKJV

MYASTHENIA GRAVIS

Great and wonderful and awe-inspiring are Your works, O Lord God, the Almighty (the Omnipotent, the Ruler of all); righteous and true are Your ways, O king of the nations! You are Alpha and Omega, the Beginning and the End, the First and the Last. You are the Good Shepherd. The good Shepherd gives His life for the sheep. I give You praise before coming to You with my concerns.

I lift my eyes to the hills from where my help comes from. My help comes from You, Lord, who made the heaven and the earth. Father, I ask that You fix the communication problem that is causing my muscles and nerves to be weak. Father, touch the antibodies that my immune system is making and unblock or change the nerve signals to my muscles, so that it will make my muscles stronger and not weaker.

Heal and restore my body from drooping eyelids, double vision, breathing issues, dysarthria (speaking), difficulty walking, distorted facial expressions, dysphagia (swallowing), and inadequate chewing. I ask that You strengthen my weakened neck, arm, and leg muscles. When I am fatigued, Father, strengthen and supply my body and mind with energy. Give me motivation so that I can perform my daily activities.

I know that some people have experienced a reduction in their symptoms by having a thymectomy. If I choose to have the thymectomy, I ask in advance, Father, that You touch the doctors, nurses, and anesthesiologist to be at their best physically and mentally. I pray that they will get enough rest, so that there will be no room for errors or mistakes during surgery. I also ask that whatever medication(s) they give me before, during, and after surgery, I will not have any side effects from them. When I go into remission, I pray that it will be permanent and not temporary, Father.

When I cry (for help), You, Lord, hear and rescue me from all my distress and troubles. When I decree a thing, it shall be established unto me. I decree and declare that my muscular, nervous, and lymphatic systems, along with my blood and immune system cells, will be in harmony with the design You established for their functionality.

According to Your Word, Jesus was wounded for my transgressions, He was bruised for my iniquities, and the chastisement of my peace was upon Him, and by His stripes, **I AM HEALED!** Death and life are in the power of the tongue, so I speak life over my body. I decree and declare prosperity of healing over my body. In Jesus' name.

Whatever medication(s) I am prescribed, I pray that I will not have any side effects and it will help me, not further harm me, in the name of Jesus. I ask that You turn my discomfort into comfort and allow me to live an active and healthy life. I cancel every assignment that Satan has for me, and I bind it up.

As Your Word states, Jesus cast out the spirits with a word and healed all that were sick. I ask in faith that You heal me completely. For whatever things I ask in prayer, believing, I will receive. I thank You for hearing and answering my prayers, Father. Thank You for being the Great Shepherd and a Miracle Worker. Amen!

{Revelation 15:3 (AMP), Revelation 22:13, John 10:11, Psalm 121:1-2,

Psalm 34:17 (AMP), Job 22:28, Isaiah 53:5, 3 John 2, Matthew 16:19, Matthew 8:16, Matthew 21:22, John 10:11, Job 5:9} NKJV

MYOSITIS

God, You are my Salvation; I will trust and not be afraid, for You, Lord, are my strength and song. I will honor and praise Your name, for You are my God. You do such wonderful things! You planned them long ago, and now You have accomplished them.

Father, You told me to cast all my cares [all my anxieties, all my worries, and all my concerns], once and for all, on You, for You care about me [with deepest affection] and watch over me very carefully. I bring before You my prayers, asking that You smother and release the inflammation in my muscles and tissues so that it won't cause further damage. Decrease and eliminate the pain and soreness in my muscles. Father, stretch forth Your healing hands towards me and help me get up out of a chair, climb stairs, lift my arms up, and grasp objects.

When I feel like I am losing my balance or start to trip, help me not to hurt myself. Touch my longitudinal pharyngeal muscles so that I can swallow easily without any difficulties. I am asking for strength in my weakened muscles, as well as when I am fatigued. For Your grace is sufficient for me; for Your strength is made perfect in my weakness.

I rather glory in my infirmities, that the power of Christ may rest upon me. For You give power to the weak and increase strength to all those who have no might. I pray that You allow the treatments that I'm taking to help speed up my recovery from the attacks of this incurable disease that I am battling. Heal me from the crown of my head to the soles of my feet.

I decree and declare that my muscular, respiratory, and digestive systems, along with my blood and immune system cells, will be in harmony with the design You established for their functionality.

According to Your Word, Jesus was wounded for my transgressions, He was bruised for my iniquities, and the chastisement of my peace was upon Him, and by His stripes, **I AM HEALED!** Death and life are in the power of the tongue, so I speak life over my body. I decree and declare prosperity of healing over my body. In Jesus' name.

Whatever medication(s) I am prescribed, I pray that I will not have

any side effects and it will help me, not further harm me, in the name of Jesus. Thank You, Father, that You have heard my prayers and seen my tears; surely You will heal me. I thank You that Your Word will not return unto You void, but it shall accomplish what You please. Thank You for being my Deliverer and my Restorer. Amen!

{Isaiah 12:2, Isaiah 25:1, 1 Peter 5:7 (AMP), 2 Corinthians 12:9, Isaiah 40:29, Job 22:28, Isaiah 53:5, Proverbs 18:21, 3 John 2, 2 Kings 20:5, Isaiah 55:11, Psalm 18:2, Psalm 23:3} NKJV

NEUROMYELITIS OPTICA (DEVIC'S DISEASE)NMO

Father, You are the Everlasting God, the Lord, the Creator of the ends of the earth, who neither faints nor is weary. Your understanding is unsearchable. You are God, and there is no other, and there is none like You. It is good to give thanks to You, Lord, and to sing praises to Your name, O Most High; I will declare Your lovingkindness in the morning and Your faithfulness every night.

I will call upon You, Lord, who is worthy to be praised. Father, Your Word states that before I call, You will answer; while I am still speaking, You will hear. I am seeking Your face, Father, asking that You heal my immune system so that it will stop mistakenly attacking the healthy cells and proteins in my body. I pray that You smother and release the inflammation in my optic nerve and spinal cord.

Decrease and eliminate the pain and spasms that I am experiencing in my eyes and muscles. Father, stop the vomiting, bladder/bowel problem, and the hiccups I am having. Strengthen me during this time of weakness and bring back the feeling from the loss of sensation that I am experiencing. Father, I ask that You touch my body so that I can have fewer cluster attacks.

I ask that the attacks will not last for months or years. I know that people have periods of remission with NMO. Father, I pray that I will go into complete remission from NMO with a permanent absence of the condition. I thank You in advance for complete healing of my central nervous system.

I decree and declare that my nervous, musculoskeletal, digestive, and urinary systems, along with my blood and immune system cells, will be in harmony with the design You established for their functionality.

According to Your Word, Jesus was wounded for my transgressions, He was bruised for my iniquities, and the chastisement of my peace was upon Him, and by His stripes, **I AM HEALED!** Death and life are in the power of the tongue, so I speak life over my body. I decree and declare prosperity of healing over my body. In Jesus' name.

Whatever medication(s) I am prescribed, I pray that I will not have any side effects and it will help me, not further harm me, in the name of Jesus. Thank You for giving me power when my body is weak from NMO and for giving me strength when I have no might, Father God. Thank You for being my Refuge and my Strength. Amen!

{Isaiah 40:28, Isaiah 46:9, Psalm 92:1-2, Psalm 118:3, Isaiah 65:24, Job 22:28, Isaiah 53:5, Job 22:28, 3 John 2, Isaiah 40:29, Psalm 46:1} NKJV

OCULAR CICATRICAL PEMPHIGOID

Lord, You are the true God; You are the living God and the Everlasting King. "Blessed be Your name, God, forever and ever, for wisdom and might are Yours." You are the All-Knowing Physician Jehovah Rapha (The Lord Who Heals) who can heal and deliver me from this disease. You are the only God I've had or ever will have; You are incomparable and irreplaceable.

Father, I come to You asking for restoration and complete healing from this rare chronic blistering and scarring disease that is affecting my oral and ocular mucosa. Decrease and eliminate the painful, oozing blisters on my skin, nose, eyes, mouth, intestinal tract, and genitals, Father. I ask with faith that You smother and release the inflammation in my conjunctiva so the discomfort, redness, dryness, and grittiness of my eyes will go away. Whatever I ask in prayer, believing, I will receive.

So, Father, I stand on Your Word and confess healing over my body. I decree and declare that my nervous, integumentary, and reproductive systems, along with my blood and immune system cells, will be in harmony with the design You established for their functionality.

According to Your Word, Jesus was wounded for my transgressions, He was bruised for my iniquities, and the chastisement of my peace was upon Him, and by His stripes, **I AM HEALED!** Death and life are in the power of the tongue, so I speak life over my body. I decree and declare prosperity of healing over my body. In Jesus' name.

Whatever medication(s) I am prescribed, I pray that I will not have any of the side effects and that it will help me, not further harm me, in the name of Jesus. I thank You, Father, that when I cry (for help), You hear and rescue me from all my distresses and troubles. Thank You for hearing the effective, fervent prayers of a righteous man/woman. Thank You for comforting me during my time of need, Father God. Amen!

{Jeremiah 10:10, Daniel 2:20, Romans 11:33, Exodus 15:26, Isaiah 46:9 (MSG),

Matthew 21:22, Job 22:28, Isaiah 53:5, Proverbs 18:21, 3 John 2, Psalm 34:17 (AMP), James 5:16b} NKJV

PALINDROMIC RHEUMATISM

God, You are the Rock and Your work is perfect; for all Your ways are justice, a God of truth without justice. Righteous and upright are You. Father, Your ways are perfect; You are a Shield to all who trust in You. Great are You, Lord, and abundant in strength. Your understanding is infinite.

I will exalt You, my God, O King, and (with gratitude and submissive wonder) I will bless Your name forever and ever. I want to bring You honor and praise before I bring my requests to You. I lift up my eyes to the hills from where my help comes from. My help comes from You, Lord, who made the heavens and the earth.

. . .

FATHER, I ask that You reduce swelling and loosen up my stiff joints. Also, smother and release the inflammation in my joints. I ask that You decrease and eliminate the pain in my hands, wrists, feet, and knees, Father. Decrease the attacks so that I will not have them for several hours or several days.

I know that some people can develop rheumatoid arthritis, so please, Father, don't let me be one of them. Hear my prayer, O Lord, and let my cry come to You. Do not hide Your face from me in the day of my trouble; incline Your ear to me; in the day that I call, answer me speedily. I ask that my healing shall spring forth speedily.

I decree and declare that my musculoskeletal system, along with my blood and immune system cells, will be in harmony with the design You established for their functionality.

According to Your Word, Jesus was wounded for my transgressions, He was bruised for my iniquities, and the chastisement of my peace was upon Him, and by His stripes, **I AM HEALED!** Death and life are in the power of the tongue, so I speak life over my body. I decree and declare prosperity of healing over my body. In Jesus' name.

Whatever medication(s) I am prescribed, I pray that I will not have any side effects and it will help me, not further harm me, in the name of Jesus. I thank You in advance for total healing, for You are the Lord Who Heals. Amen!

{Deuteronomy 32:4, Psalm 18:30, Psalm 147:5, Psalm 145:1 (AMP), Psalm 121:1-2, Psalm 102:1, Isaiah 58:8a, Job 22:28, Isaiah 53:5, Proverbs 18:21, 3 John 2, Exodus 14:26} NKJV

PAROXYSMAL NOCTURNAL HEMOGLOBINURIA (PNH)

Blessed be the name of God forever and ever, for wisdom and might are Yours. Ah, Lord God! Behold, You have made the heavens and the earth by Your great power and outstretched arm. There is nothing too hard for You, God.

You are good, Lord, a stronghold in the day of trouble, and You know those who trust in You. Father, You are the All-Knowing

Physician Jehovah Rapha (The Lord Who Heals), who can heal and deliver me from this rare, acquired disorder that leads to premature death of my blood cells. Father, before I call, You will answer; while I am still speaking, You will hear my prayers. I come to You asking that You touch my red blood cells and allow them not to break down prematurely so the hemoglobin won't leak into my blood, which can pass into my urine.

Father, reverse the defective blood cells in my body so that they can produce normal, effective cells. I know that this disorder can cause severe bone marrow dysfunction. I'm asking that You increase my low levels of red and white blood cells, along with my platelets, so that I will not form blood clots. Father, decrease and eliminate the pain from the associated headaches, chest pains, and abdominal contractions.

Give me strength when I'm fatigued. Take away the shortness of breath, fever, chronic renal disease, and bruising/bleeding underneath my skin. I believe that You can heal me, Father, because not only did Jesus preach the gospel in Galilee, but He also healed all kinds of sicknesses and diseases among the people. If You can do it for them, I know You can do it for me because You do not have partiality, Father.

Your Word tells me that whatever things I ask in prayer, believing, I will receive. I decree and declare that my urinary, renal, cardiovascular, digestive, and respiratory systems, along with my blood and immune system cells, will be in harmony with the design You established for their functionality.

According to Your Word, Jesus was wounded for my transgressions, He was bruised for my iniquities, and the chastisement of my peace was upon Him, and by His stripes, **I AM HEALED!** Death and life are in the power of the tongue, so I speak life over my body. I decree and declare prosperity of healing over my body. In Jesus' name.

Whatever medication(s) I am prescribed, I pray that I will not have any side effects and it will help me, not further harm me, in the name of Jesus. I thank You that my healing shall spring forth speedily, for You are the Lord Who Heals and will restore my health from this disorder. Amen!

{Daniel 2:20, Jeremiah 32:17, Nahum 1:7, Exodus 15:26, Isaiah 65:24, Matthew 4:23, Romans 2:11, Matthew 21:22, Job 22:28, Isaiah 53:5, Proverbs 18:21, 3 John 2, Isaiah 58:8a, Exodus 14:26} NKJV

PARSONAGE-TURNER SYNDROME (PTS)

Father, You are a good shepherd. A Shepherd who gives His life for me. You existed before all things, and in You, all things consist (cohere, held together). God, please bend an ear to my prayer concerning this uncommon neurological autoimmune disorder. As I call out to You, guide me up High Rock Mountain. As for You, Father, Your ways are perfect: the Word of the Lord is tried: You are the buckler to all those that trust in You. All praises go to You.

Father, You told me to cast all my cares upon You, for You care for me. Your Word says, come to me all who labor and are heavy laden, and I will give you rest. I am seeking Your help. I'm asking for healing and restoration from this neurological disorder. Father, I ask that You decrease and eliminate the severe and intense pain that I am experiencing in my upper arms, shoulders, forearms, and/or hands. I ask that You touch my motor nerves and axons so that they can function the way You made them, without muscle weakness.

Allow my weakened muscles to regain their strength and functionality so that I can perform my daily activities. I decree and declare that my musculoskeletal and nervous systems, along with immune cells, will be in harmony with the design You established for their functionality.

According to Your Word, Jesus was wounded for my transgressions, He was bruised for my iniquities, and the chastisement of my peace was upon Him, and by His stripes, **I AM HEALED!** Death and life are in the power of the tongue, so I speak life over my body. I decree and declare prosperity of healing over my body. In Jesus' name.

Whatever medication(s) I am prescribed, I pray that I will not have any side effects and it will help me, not further harm me, in the name

of Jesus. I cancel every assignment that Satan has over my health and call it ineffective. I trust and believe that You will heal, deliver, strengthen, and restore my body from the crown of my head to the very soles of my feet. You are the God whose Word will not return unto You void but shall accomplish what You please.

I thank You that You have heard my prayer and You have seen my tears; surely You will heal me, Father. Thank You, Father, for being my Restorer. Amen!

{John 10:11, Colossians 1:17 (AMPC), Psalm 61:2 (MSG), Psalm 18:30, 1 Peter 5:7, Matthew 11:28, Job 22:28, Isaiah 53:5, Proverbs 18:21, 3 John 2, Isaiah 55:11, 2 Kings 20:5, Psalm 23:3} NKJV

PEMPHIGUS VULGARIS

God, You are good to one and all; everything You do is soaked through with grace. It is because of Your lovingkindness that I am not consumed because Your tender compassions never fail. They are new every morning; great and beyond measure is Your faithfulness, Lord. I come lifting up my eyes to the hills from where my help comes from. My help comes from You, Father.

I'm asking for relief from the painful blisters and erosions on my skin and mucus membranes. Father, I ask that You decrease and dissolve the blisters in my mouth, throat, and genitals so that it will not be difficult to eat and swallow. Touch my skin that has open sore(s) and shield them from becoming infected.

(For the ones battling with an infection, add this to your prayer) Father, I ask that You stop and take away the infection in my skin and do not allow it to spread to my bloodstream, causing me to have sepsis. Stretch forth Your healing hands and turn my discomfort to comfort, for my desire is to be pain-free and blister-free, Father. When I cry (for help), Lord, You hear and rescue me from all my distress and troubles.

I decree and declare that my integumentary, digestive, and

reproduction systems, along with blood and immune cells, will be in harmony with the design You established for their functionality.

According to Your Word, Jesus was wounded for my transgressions, He was bruised for my iniquities, and the chastisement of my peace was upon Him, and by His stripes, **I AM HEALED!** Death and life are in the power of the tongue, so I speak life over my body. I decree and declare prosperity of healing over my body. In Jesus' name.

Whatever medication(s) I am prescribed, I pray that I will not have any side effects and it will help me, not further harm me, in the name of Jesus. I thank You, Everlasting God, that my healing shall spring forth speedily. You are the God who does wonders; You have declared Your strength among the peoples. Amen!

{Psalm 145:9 (MSG), Lamentations 3:22-23 (AMP), Psalm 121:1-2, Psalm 34:17 (AMP), Job 22:28, Isaiah 53:5, Proverbs 18:21, 3 John 2, Isaiah 40:28, Isaiah 58:8a, Psalm 77:14} NKJV

POEMS SYNDROME (POLYNEUROPATHY, ORGANOMEGALY, ENDOCRINOPATHY, MONOCLONAL GAMMOPATHY, SKIN CHANGES)

Great and wonderful and awe-inspiring are Your works, O Lord God, the Almighty (Omnipotent, the Ruler of all); righteous and true are Your ways, O King of the nations! I praise You, Lord, for You are good; I sing praises to Your name, for it is pleasant. I thank You, Father, that I am complete in You, who is the head of all principality and power. You are not a man, that You should lie, nor a son of man, that You should repent.

You spoke it, and You will make good on Your promise. Your Word shall not return unto You void, but it shall accomplish what You please. You have never left me nor forsaken me, and You won't start now. I'm bringing before You this rare multisystem disorder that damages my nerves and other body parts.

With this disorder, there is a lot going on in my body, Father. Touch my body and take away the numbness and tingling in my hands, toes, feet, and legs. Decrease and eliminate the pain, as well as smother and release the inflammation in the affected areas. Shrink my spleen, liver, and/or lymph nodes down to the size You made them to be.

Father, balance my hormone levels so that they won't continue to cause me to have an underactive thyroid, fatigue, diabetes, sexual issues, swelling in my limbs, and other necessary functions. Turn my bone marrow cells back to normal so that they will not continue to produce protein in my bloodstream. Decrease the thickness of my skin, facial and leg hair, along with returning my skin color to the way You made me. Send Your Word, Father, and heal me.

I decree and declare that my lymphatic, endocrine, integumentary, nervous, respiratory, and circulatory systems, along with my endothelial, contractile, blood and immune cells, will be in harmony with the design You established for their functionality.

According to Your Word, Jesus was wounded for my transgressions, He was bruised for my iniquities, and the chastisement of my peace was upon Him, and by His stripes, **I AM HEALED!** Death and life are in the power of the tongue, so I speak life over my body. I decree and declare prosperity of healing over my body. In Jesus' name.

Whatever medication(s) I am prescribed, I pray that I will not have any side effects and it will help me, not further harm me, in the name of Jesus. I thank You in advance, Father, for healing, deliverance, and restoration in my body. I will continue to lean on and trust in You, All-Powerful God, for there is nothing too hard for You. I thank You that You have heard my prayers, You have seen my tears; surely You will heal me. Amen!

{Revelation 15:3 (AMP), Psalm 135:3, Colossians 2:10, Numbers 23:19 (AMP), Isaiah 55:11, Deuteronomy 31:6, Psalm 107:20, Job 22:28, Isaiah 53:5, Proverbs 18:21, 3 John 2, Proverbs 3:5, Jeremiah 32:17, 2 Kings 20:5} NKJV

POLYARTERITIS NODOSA (PAN)

Who will not fear (reverently) and glorify Your name, O Lord (giving You honor and praise in worship)? For You alone are Holy; for all the nations shall come and worship before You, for Your righteous acts (Your just decrees and judgments) have been revealed and displayed. You are Alpha and Omega, the Beginning and the End, the First and the Last. I praise You, God, for Your mighty acts; I praise You according to Your excellent greatness!

Thank You, Father, for allowing Your son, Jesus Christ, to take my infirmities and bear my sickness. You are the source of all healing. I put my trust in You that You can and will strengthen, heal, and restore my body from this serious autoimmune-related blood vessel disease.

Smother and release the inflammation of the blood vessels so that it can no longer restrict blood from flowing and causing damage to my vital organs and tissues. Decrease and eliminate the pain in my abdomen, joints, muscles, chest, skin sores and (testicular in men). Strengthen me when I am fatigued and comfort me. Regulate my blood pressure, so that it won't cause my kidney any damage.

I know with this disease, there is a high risk for an aneurysm to occur. I am asking now, in advance, that You protect my artery wall so that this will not happen to me. I decree and declare that my nervous, integumentary, urinary, circulatory, musculoskeletal, and digestive systems, along with blood and immune system cells, will be in harmony with the design You established for their functionality.

According to Your Word, Jesus was wounded for my transgressions, He was bruised for my iniquities, and the chastisement of my peace was upon Him, and by His stripes, **I AM HEALED!** Death and life are in the power of the tongue, so I speak life over my body. I decree and declare prosperity of healing over my body. In Jesus' name.

Whatever medication(s) I am prescribed, I pray that I will not have any side effects and it will help me, not further harm me, in the name of Jesus. I thank You for restoring my health and for healing my wounds, Father. Thank You for answering my prayers, for the effective, fervent prayers of a righteous man avails much. Thank You for being the God of Hope and the God of My Life. Amen!

{**Revelation 15:4 (AMP), Revelation 22:13, Psalm 150:2, Matthew 8:17, Job 22:28, Isaiah 53:5, Proverbs 18:21, 3 John 2, Jeremiah 30:17, James 5:16b, Romans 15:18, Psalm 42:8**} NKJV

POLYMYALGIA RHEUMATICA

You are the Root and the Offspring of David, the Bright and Morning Star, Jesus. You are worthy, O Lord, to receive glory and honor and power, for You created all things, and by Your will, they exist and were created. I know that the Lord lives! Blessed be my Rock!

I will exalt You, Father, for You are the Rock of my salvation! I will sing to You, Lord; I will sing praises to You, Lord God of Israel. I will call upon You, Lord, for You are worthy to be praised. Now that I have given You praise, I am casting all my cares [all my anxieties, all my worries, and all my concerns], once and for all, on You, for You care about me [with deepest affection] and watch over me very carefully.

Father, I ask that You decrease and eliminate the widespread pain and stiffness that I am experiencing, especially in the mornings. Strengthen my body from being fatigued and take away the malaise. Help me commit to the exercises that were given to me so that I will have strength in the areas that have limited range of motion. I decree and declare that my musculoskeletal system, along with my blood and immune system cells, will be in harmony with the design You established for their functionality.

According to Your Word, Jesus was wounded for my transgressions, He was bruised for my iniquities, and the chastisement of my peace was upon Him, and by His stripes, **I AM HEALED!** Death and life are in the power of the tongue, so I speak life over my body. I decree and declare prosperity of healing over my body. In Jesus' name.

Whatever medication(s) I am prescribed, I pray that I will not have

any side effects and it will help me, not further harm me, in the name of Jesus.

I believe that You can and will heal me. Jesus healed many people who were sick with various diseases, and if He can do it for them, I know He can do it for me. One thing about You, Father, there is no partiality with You. I thank You in advance for springing forth my healing speedily. Thank You for being the Everlasting Father and the God of all Comfort. Amen!

{Revelation 22:16, Revelation 4:11, 2 Samuel 22:47, Judges 5:3, 1 Peter 5:7 (AMP), Job 22:28, Isaiah 53:5, Proverbs 18:21, 3 John 2, Mark 1:34, Romans 2:11, Isaiah 58:8a, 2 Corinthians 1:3} NKJV

POLYMYOSITIS

I want to give You honor and praise before I bring You my concerns. Holy, holy, holy, are You, Lord God, the Almighty (the Omnipotent, the Ruler of all), who was, who is, and who is to come (the unchanging, eternal God). Father, You are my strength and song, and You have become my salvation; You are God, and I will praise and exalt You. You are the Rock; Your work is perfect; for all Your ways are justice, a God of truth and without injustice; Righteous and upright are You, Father.

I lift my eyes up to the hills from where my help comes from. My help comes from You, Lord, who made heaven and earth. Father, stretch forth Your healing hands and stop the inflammatory cells from directly attacking the muscle fibers in my immune system so that I won't continue to have this systemic disease. Heal my muscles that are damaged from this disease.

I ask that You smother and release the inflammation in my muscles so that it won't cause any further damage to my muscles or associated tissues. Decrease and eliminate the pain in my upper arms, neck, shoulders, thighs, and hips. Strengthen my weakened muscles so that I can get out of bed and perform my daily tasks. Help me commit to doing the exercises that are prescribed so that I won't lose range of motion.

Heal me completely so that I will not have any flare-ups. If I do, please don't let them be acute, so I don't have to use a walker, cane, or wheelchair. Father, protect my respiratory, heart, and esophagus from becoming affected by this disease.

(For the ones that have their heart, respiratory, and esophagus affected, add this to your prayer) Father, smother and release the inflammation in my lung tissues, along with my heart muscles, and heal them from any damage this disease has caused.

Touch my esophagus with Your healing hands and alleviate my swallowing difficulties, and touch my lungs to enhance my breathing problems. Heal my heart to eliminate the chances of a heart attack, stroke, heart failure, or the requirement for a heart transplant, Father. I decree and declare that my musculoskeletal, respiratory, and cardiovascular systems, along with my blood and immune cells, will be in harmony with the design You established for their functionality.

According to Your Word, Jesus was wounded for my transgressions, He was bruised for my iniquities, and the chastisement of my peace was upon Him, and by His stripes, **I AM HEALED!** Death and life are in the power of the tongue, so I speak life over my body. I decree and declare prosperity of healing over my body. In Jesus' name.

Whatever medication(s) I am prescribed, I pray that I will not have any side effects and it will help me, not further harm me, in the name of Jesus. I thank You that my prayer of faith will restore me. Before I call, You will answer; while I am still speaking, You will hear my prayers for healing, Father. I believe that You can and will strengthen, heal, and restore my body. I put my healing in Your hands, Father. Amen!

{Revelation 4:8 (AMP), Exodus 15:2, Deuteronomy 32:4, Psalm 121:1-2, Job 22:28, Isaiah 53:5, Proverbs 18:21, 3 John 2, Isaiah 65:24}

PRIMARY BILIARY CIRRHOSIS (PBS)

Father, I come to You with praise on my lips. You are A to Z. You are the God who is, the God who was, and the God who is about to arrive. You are the Sovereign-Strong God.

I will thank and praise You, Lord, every morning and every evening. You are my why. You are my God, who has done great and awesome things which my eyes have seen. You are good, and Your mercy endures forever. You are a good Father, and your love for me never fails.

You are the source of all healing, Father. I pray that You smother and release the inflammation in the bile ducts of my liver. Father, stop my skin from being itchy and give me strength when I am fatigued. Touch my mouth so that I will make sufficient salivary secretion, so that my mouth will not be dry.

Touch my lacrimal gland so that it can make enough tears and relieve the dryness that I am experiencing. Decrease and eliminate the pain in my right upper abdomen, joints, muscles, and bones. **(Add other symptoms that you are having that are not listed.)** Stretch forth Your healing hands and allow me to make enough bile so that my digestive system will have the ability to absorb fats and the fat-soluble vitamins A, D, E, and K.

Father, protect my body from having further complications, like liver cancer, enlarged spleen, enlarged veins, and/or osteoporosis. I decree and declare my digestive, musculoskeletal, nervous, and integumentary system, along with blood and immune system cells, will be in harmony with the design You established for their functionality.

According to Your Word, Jesus was wounded for my transgressions, He was bruised for my iniquities, and the chastisement of my peace was upon Him, and by His stripes **I AM HEALED!** Death and life are in the power of the tongue, so I speak life over my body. I decree and declare prosperity of healing over my body. In Jesus' name.

Whatever medication(s) I am prescribed, I pray that I will not have any side effects and it will help me, not further harm me, in the name

of Jesus. My trust is in You, and I thank You in advance for my complete and total healing, Everlasting God. Thank You that Your Word shall not return unto You void but shall accomplish what You please. Amen!

{Revelation 1:8 (MSG), 1 Chronicles 23:30, Deuteronomy 10:21, 2 Chronicles 7:3, Job 22:28, Isaiah 53:5, Proverbs 18:21, 3 John 2, Isaiah 9:6, Isaiah 55:11} NKJV

PRIMARY SCLEROSING CHOLANGITIS (PSC)

Lord God, there is no God in heaven above or on earth below like You, who keeps Your covenant and mercy with Your servants, who walk before You with all their hearts. I will praise You, Lord, according to Your righteousness and will sing praise to the name of the Lord Most High. I give thanks to You, Lord, for You are good! Father, You do great things and unsearchable, marvelous things without number.

I rejoice in You, Lord, O You Righteous! For praise from the upright is beautiful. I lift up my eyes to the hills from where my help comes. My help comes from You, Lord, who made heaven and earth.

Before I call, You will answer. While I am still speaking, You will hear my prayers. Father, I ask that You smother and release the inflammation in my bile ducts so–that it will not continue to cause further scarring and destruction of my liver cells. I pray that I have none or little to no scar tissue so that the drainage of my bile ducts will not be blocked and cause me to have an infection. Father, dissolve the itching, yellow eyes/skin, abdominal pain, and fatigue.

Help me to submit and commit to the changes that are needed, so that I can preserve my liver function. I can do this with Your help because my help comes from You. I ask that the disease does not worsen over time and cause me to have liver failure, requiring a transplant.

(For those on the transplant list, this prayer is for you) Father, I know that there are other people on the transplant list who need a liver like I do. I ask not out of selfishness, but that I will find favor in Your eyes and in the eyes of man, so that I will be one of the ones that will receive a liver. I also ask that the other people on the list receive one as well. Father, You are the source of all healing.

I decree and declare my digestive, muscular, nervous, and integumentary system, along with my blood and immune system cells, will be in harmony with the design You established for their functionality.

According to Your Word, Jesus was wounded for my transgressions, He was bruised for my iniquities, and the chastisement of my peace was upon Him, and by His stripes, **I AM HEALED!** Death and life are in the power of the tongue, so I speak life over my body. I decree and declare prosperity of healing over my body. In Jesus' name.

Whatever medication(s) I am prescribed, I pray that I will not have any side effects and it will help me, not further harm me, in the name of Jesus. Stretch forth Your hand towards me and regenerate my liver, for You are the Giver of Life. Amen!

{1 Kings 8:23, 1 Chronicles 16:34, Psalm 33:1, Psalm 121:1-2, Isaiah 65:24, Job 22:28, Isaiah 53:5, Proverbs 18:21, 3 John 2, Job 33:4} NKJV

PSORIASIS

I want to give You what's due to You first, Father, and that is praise and worship. I will praise You, O Lord, with my whole heart; I will tell of all Your marvelous works. I will be glad and rejoice in You; I will sing praises to Your name, O Most High. You do great things (beyond understanding), unfathomable, yes, marvelous, and wonderous things without number. You are my Strength and my Shield; my heart trusts in You, and I am helped; therefore, my heart greatly rejoices, and with song I will praise You.

I come boldly to the throne of grace that I might obtain mercy and find grace in my time of help. I am seeking comfort from the itching that I am experiencing in my knees, elbows, face, scalp, feet, and palms. Turn my discomfort to comfort, Father. Decrease and eliminate the soreness and stinging on my skin.

Father, I ask that You slow down my overactive immune system so that my skin cells will go through the normal growth and shedding process. Protect my healthy tissues and organs from any further damage from this disease. Your Word states that whatever things I ask in prayer, believing, I will receive. I believe and trust in You, Father, that You can and will heal, strengthen, and restore my body.

I decree and declare that my integumentary and musculoskeletal systems, along with my blood and immune system cells, will be in harmony with the design You established for their functionality.

According to Your Word, Jesus was wounded for my transgressions, He was bruised for my iniquities, and the chastisement of my peace was upon Him, and by His stripes, **I AM HEALED!** Death and life are in the power of the tongue, so I speak life over my body. I decree and declare prosperity of healing over my body. In Jesus' name.

Whatever medication(s) I am prescribed, I pray that I will not have any side effects and it will help me, not further harm me, in the name of Jesus.

Thank You for allowing me to cast all my cares upon You, Father, for You care for me. Thank You that You are not a man who does not lie. You are not human, so You do not change Your mind. Have You ever spoken and failed to act? You have never made a promise and not carried it through. Thank You that my healing shall spring forth speedily. Amen!

{Psalm 9:1-2, Job 9:10 (AMP), Psalm 28:7, Hebrews 4:16, Matthew 21:22, Job 22:28, Isaiah 53:5, Proverbs 18:21, 3 John 2, 1 Peter 5:7, Numbers 23:19 (AMP), Isaiah 58:8a} NKJV

PSORIATIC ARTHRITIS

Blessed are You, Lord God of Israel, our Father, forever and ever. Yours, O Lord, is the greatness, the power, the glory, the victory, and the majesty; for all that is in heaven and in earth is Yours; Yours is the kingdom, O LORD, and You are exalted as head overall. Both riches and honor come from You, and You reign overall. In Your hands is power and might; in Your hands, it is to make great and to give strength to all.

Now, therefore, our God, we thank You and praise Your glorious name. Father, You told me to cast all my cares [all my anxieties, all my worries, and all my concerns, once and for all] on You, for You care about me [with deepest affection and watch over me very carefully]. Father, I'm asking for strength, healing, deliverance, and restoration from this chronic form of arthritis that is attacking my skin, small/large joints, organs, and spine. Smother and release the inflammation in my joints, fingers, toes, spine, and eyes.

Loosen my stiff joints and reverse the fatigue so I can have energy like never before. Father, decrease and eliminate the pain in my joints, spine, foot, and eyes. Stop my immune system from fighting itself and protect my healthy tissues from further damage from this disease. I decree and declare that my integumentary and musculoskeletal systems, along with blood and immune system cells, will be in harmony with the design You established for their functionality.

According to Your Word, Jesus was wounded for my transgressions, He was bruised for my iniquities, and the chastisement of my peace was upon Him, and by His stripes, **I AM HEALED!** Death and life are in the power of the tongue, so I speak life over my body. I decree and declare prosperity of healing over my body. In Jesus' name.

Whatever medication(s) I am prescribed, I pray that I will not have any side effects and it will help me, not further harm me, in the name of Jesus. I pray that I will not have any flare-ups, but if I do, I ask for God's healing speedily.

In my distress, I called upon You, Lord, and cried out to You; You heard my voice from Your temple, and my cry came before Your ears. Thank You for being my Refuge and my Strength, Father. Amen!

{1 Chronicles 29:11-13, 1 Peter 5:7 (AMP), Job 22:28, Isaiah 53:5, Proverbs 18:21, 3 John 2, Psalms 18:6, Psalm 46:1} NKJV

PURE RED CELL APLASIA (PRCA)

Blessed be Your glorious name, which is exalted above all blessing and praise! You alone are the Lord; You have made heaven, the heaven of heavens, with all their host, the earth and everything on it. The seas and all that is in them, and You preserve them all. The host of heaven worships You.

I will sing praises to Your name, Lord God. I want to enter into Your gates with thanksgiving and into Your courts with praise. I am thankful to You and will bless Your name. I am seeking You for strength and healing from this bone marrow disorder.

Touch my bone marrow and cause it to make an adequate amount of red blood cells so the fatigue, difficulty breathing, pale skin, and dizziness can go away. I know that this disorder can be inherited, acquired, or induced by medication. If I inherited it, I pray that it will cease with me and that it will not pass on to my children. If there is a medication(s) that I am taking that causes me to have this disorder, replace it with a medication(s) that will not cause this.

If this disorder arises as a consequence of another disorder/disease, I ask that You heal every affected area of my body, Father. Give me energy when I am fatigued and lethargic. Strengthen my body, for Your grace is sufficient for me, and Your strength is made perfect in weakness. I decree and declare my circulatory, skeletal, respiratory, integumentary, and endocrine systems, along with my blood and immune system cells, will be in harmony with the design You established for their functionality.

According to Your Word, Jesus was wounded for my transgressions, He was bruised for my iniquities, and the chastisement of my peace was upon Him, and by His stripes, **I AM HEALED!** Death and life are in the power of the tongue, so I speak life over my body. I decree and declare prosperity of healing over my body. In Jesus' name.

Whatever medication(s) I am prescribed, I pray that I will not have any side effects and it will help me, not further harm me, in the name

of Jesus. I thank You in advance for total healing. Thank You for being the Lord who is always there for me when I need You. Amen!

{**Nehemiah 9:5-6, Judges 5:3, Psalm 100:4, 2 Corinthians 12:9, Job 22:28, Isaiah 53:5, Proverbs 18:21, 3 John 2, Ezekiel 48:35} NKJV**

PYODERMA GANGRENOSUM

Before I cast my cares upon You, Father, I want to brag on You first. You do great things and unsearchable, marvelous things without number. You have made me, and the breath of the Almighty gives me life. I will praise You, Lord, according to Your righteousness and will sing praises to Your name Most High.

Therefore, by You, Father, I will continually offer the sacrifice of praise to You, God, that is the fruit of my lips, giving thanks to Your name. I come to You, Father, with my plea, asking that You take away these painful ulcers. Decrease and eliminate the pain. I come boldly to the throne of grace that I may obtain mercy and find grace for help in a time of need. I ask for a Godspeed recovery from this rare inflammatory skin disorder.

Smother and release the inflammation in my body. Decrease and release the pain from the ulcer(s) that I have. Close up the open sore(s) and protect them from possible complications of infection, scarring, and/or mobility loss. If this disorder is linked to any other systemic disease(s) that I have, I ask that You heal every part of my body that is being impacted.

When I cry out for help, Lord, You hear and rescue me from all my distress and troubles. I decree and declare that my integumentary and circulatory systems, along with my blood and immune system cells, will be in harmony with the design You established for their functionality.

According to Your Word, Jesus was wounded for my transgressions, He was bruised for my iniquities, and the chastisement of my peace was upon Him, and by His stripes, **I AM HEALED!** Death and life are in the power of the tongue, so I speak life over my

body. I decree and declare prosperity of healing over my body. In Jesus' name.

Whatever medication(s) I am prescribed, I pray that I will not have any side effects and it will help me, not further harm me, in the name of Jesus. I know that this disease may leave some scarring, Father. So, every time I see the scar, I will think of Your goodness and how You healed me. I give thanks to You, Lord of Lords!

For Your mercy endures forever. I thank You, Father, that You are the source of my healing. Amen!

{Job 5:9, Job 33:4, Psalm 7:17, Hebrews 13:15, Hebrews 4:16, Psalm 34:17 (AMP), Job 22:28, Isaiah 53:5, Proverbs 18:21, 3 John 2, Psalm 136:3} NKJV

RAYNAUD'S PHENOMENON

I come before Your presence with thanksgiving; I shout joyfully to You with psalms. O Lord, I will honor and praise Your name, for You are my God. You do such wonderful things! You planned them long ago, and now you have accomplished them.

Now to the King eternal, immortal, invisible, to You Father God who alone is wise, be honor and glory forever and ever. In every situation (no matter the circumstances), I will be thankful and continually give thanks to You, God, for this is the will of God for me in Christ Jesus. I will give thanks and praise You, O Lord my God, with all my heart, and will glorify Your name forever.

Father, You told me to cast all my cares [all my anxieties, all my worries, and all my concerns], once and for all, on You, for You care about me [with deepest affection], and You watch over me very carefully.

I bring before You my plea, asking that You widen the narrowing of my arteries so that they carry blood from my heart to other parts of my body. Increase my blood flow so the vasospasm attacks will stop in my fingers, toes, and nose. I know that I cannot avoid the cold temperatures when I'm away from my home. So, I ask that while I am out, please let the vasospasm attacks be minimal so my fingers, toes, ears, and nose will not get cold, change colors, throb, or hurt.

At times, it is very hard to do things with my hands and even difficult to walk due to the ulcerations and/or infections on my fingers and toes. I ask that You kill the infection at the root, Father. Smother and release the inflammation in my fingers and toes. Decrease and eliminate the painful, slow-healing sores on my fingertips.

Father, I ask that You increase the oxygen to my tissues so that it will not result in gangrene in my fingers and toes. I know that stress is another factor that can cause me to have spasms. So, Father, help me stay calm and stress-free and not allow myself to have any emotional upsets. When I get emotional, remind me to call on You for peace.

Your peace is nothing to be compared to because Your peace surpasses all understanding and will guard my heart and mind through Christ Jesus. With the authority You have given me in Christ Jesus, I bind up this disease and any other disease associated with Raynaud's. Whatever I bind on earth will be bound in heaven, and whatever I loose on earth will be loosed in heaven. I decree and declare my circulatory, integumentary, and nervous systems, along with my blood and immune system cells, will be in harmony with the design You established for their functionality.

According to Your Word, Jesus was wounded for my transgressions, He was bruised for my iniquities, and the chastisement of my peace was upon Him, and by His stripes, **I AM HEALED!** Death and life are in the power of the tongue, so I speak life over my body. I decree and declare prosperity of healing over my body. In Jesus' name.

Whatever medication(s) I am prescribed, I pray that I will not have any side effects and it will help me, not further harm me, in the name of Jesus. Before I call, You will answer; while I am still speaking, You will hear. You have heard my prayer; You have seen my tears; surely You will heal me, Father. I thank You in advance that my health shall spring forth speedily. You are a Great God and a Great King above all gods. Amen!

{Psalm 95:2, Isaiah 26:1 (NLT), 1 Timothy 1:17, 1 Thessalonians 5:18 (AMP),

Psalm 86:12 (AMP), 1 Peter 5:17 (AMP), Philippians 4:7, Matthew 16:19, Job 22:28, Isaiah 53:5, Proverbs 18:21, 3 John 2, Isaiah 65:24, 2 Kings 20:5, Isaiah 58:8a, Psalm 95:3} NKJV

REACTIVE ARTHRITIS

I will sing to You, Lord, a new song! For You, Lord, are great beyond description and greatly to be praised. I worship only You, Lord! Because Your loving-kindness is better than life, my lips shall praise You.

Thus, I will bless You while I live; I will lift up my hands in Your name. I want to give You praise before asking anything of You, Father. I thank You for Your son, Jesus, for allowing Him to take my infirmities and bear my sicknesses. I believe that Jesus healed all kinds of sicknesses and diseases among the people in Galilee. I also believe that You can heal me as well from this inflammatory arthritis.

I ask that You clear up whatever infection is in my bloodstream that is causing me to have Reactive Arthritis. Smother and release the inflammation in my joints, tendons, lower back, and spine. Decrease and eliminate the pain in my eyes, heels, lower back, buttock, joints, and when I urinate.

Touch me so that I will not be one of the ones who will have long, chronic, or severe arthritis because of this disease. Protect my joints so this disease won't cause any damage in any way. Thank You for allowing me to bring You my cares, for You care for me, Father. I decree and declare my skeletal, urinary, integumentary, nervous, and reproductive systems, along with my blood and immune system cells, will be in harmony with the design You established for their functionality.

According to Your Word, Jesus was wounded for my transgressions, He was bruised for my iniquities, and the chastisement of my peace was upon Him, and by His stripes, **I AM HEALED!** Death and life are in the power of the tongue, so I speak life over my

body. I decree and declare prosperity of healing over my body. In Jesus' name.

Whatever medication(s) I am prescribed, I pray that I will not have any side effects and it will help me, not further harm me, in the name of Jesus. When the righteous cry (for help), You hear and rescue us from all our distress and troubles.

Thank You, God, for hearing and answering my prayers. Thank You for being my Healer, Father. Amen!

{Psalm 96:1, Psalm 96:4 (AMP), Psalm 63:3-4, Matthew 8:17, Matthew 4:23, Job 22:28, Isaiah 53:5, Proverbs 18:21, 3 John 2, Psalm 34:17 (AMP), Exodus 15:26} NKJV

RELAPSING POLYCHONDRITIS

I enter into Your gates with thanksgiving and into Your courts with praise. I am thankful to You, Lord, and I will bless Your name. You are my Strength and my Shield; my heart trusted in You, and I am helped; therefore, my heart greatly rejoices, and with my song I will praise You. I will praise Your great and awesome name, for You are holy.

I give You all the praises that are due to You, Father. Before I call, You will answer; while I am still speaking, You will hear me. In my distress, I called upon You, Lord, and cried out to You; You heard my voice from Your temple, and my cry came before You, even to Your ears. Father, I'm bringing my concerns to You and seeking healing from this rare and degenerative disease.

I ask that You smother and release the inflammation in my ears and joints. Decrease and eliminate the pain in my nose, eyes, ears, joints, ribs, neck, throat, and lesions on my skin. Relieve me of the general discomfort of hoarseness, shortness of breath, coughing, dizziness, and overall illness. Father, stop my immune system from targeting my cartilage so it doesn't develop further complications in my body.

Thank You for sustaining me in this battle and for complete healing from this painful and possibly life-threatening disease. I know that with this disease, I am seeing now or will have to see a rheumatologist, ophthalmologist, cardiologist, dermatologist, plastic surgeon, neurologist, otolaryngologist, and/or nephrologist. I ask that You give them wisdom, knowledge, and understanding on how to treat me and what medication(s) will work best for me. Thank You for giving me the authority to speak to my condition.

I decree and declare my nervous, integumentary, respiratory, musculoskeletal, and circulatory systems, along with my blood and immune system cells, will be in harmony with the design You established for their functionality.

According to Your Word, Jesus was wounded for my transgressions, He was bruised for my iniquities, and the chastisement of my peace was upon Him, and by His stripes, **I AM HEALED!** Death and life are in the power of the tongue, so I speak life over my body. I decree and declare prosperity of healing over my body. In Jesus' name.

Whatever medication(s) I am prescribed, I pray that I will not have any side effects and it will help me, not further harm me, in the name of Jesus. Thanks be unto You, God, who gives me victory through Christ Jesus. I will get through these tough times because I am more than a conqueror. You are Faithful and True, Father, and I put my total trust in You. Amen!

{Psalm 100:4, Psalm 28:7, Psalm 99:3, Isaiah 65:24, Psalm 18:6, Luke 10:19, Job 22:28, Isaiah 53:5, Proverbs 18:21, 3 John 2, 1 Corinthians 15:57, Romans 8:37, Revelation 19:11} NKJV

RETROPERITONEAL FIBROSIS

Bless the Lord, O my soul; and all that is within me, I will bless Your holy name! Bless the Lord, O my soul! O Lord my God, You are very great: You are clothed with honor and majesty. I will sing to You, Lord, as long as I live; I will sing praises to You, my God, while I have my being.

You will show me the path of life; in Your presence is fullness of joy; at Your right hand are pleasures forevermore. All praises go to You first before I come to You with my request. Father, Your Word tells me that whatever I ask in prayer, believing, I will receive. I ask that You decrease and remove the mass(es) in the back of my abdomen so that it will not continue to block my tubes (ureters).

Allow my urine to be carried from my kidneys to my bladder properly so that I will not continue to have this disorder. Decrease and eliminate the pain that I am having in my abdomen and legs. Smother and release the swelling and inflammation in my limbs and scrotum **(MEN)**. Increase my urine output and stop the vomiting, nausea, itching, and weight loss, Father.

I ask that You protect my kidneys from having temporary damage or kidney failure. Father, You are good to those who wait hopefully and expectantly for You, to those who seek You. I will quietly hope for Your help, God. I decree and declare that my urinary and digestive systems, along with blood and immune system cells, will be in harmony with the design You established for their functionality.

According to Your Word, Jesus was wounded for my transgressions, He was bruised for my iniquities, and the chastisement of my peace was upon Him, and by His stripes, **I AM HEALED!** Death and life are in the power of the tongue, so I speak life over my body. I decree and declare prosperity of healing over my body. In Jesus' name.

Whatever medication(s) I am prescribed, I pray that I will not have any side effects and it will help me, not further harm me, in the name of Jesus. I thank You, Father, that You rescue and protect those who love and trust in Your name. When they call on You, You will answer.

I thank You in advance for hearing and answering my plea concerning this disorder, Father. Thank You for keeping Your word, Father God. You are not a man, so You do not lie. You are not human, so You don't change Your mind. You have spoken and never failed to act. You have promised and will carry it through. Amen!

{Psalm 103:1, Psalm 104:1, Psalm 104:33, Psalm 16:11, Matthew 21:22,

Lamentations 3:25 (AMPC), Lamentations 3:26 (MSG), Job 22:28, Isaiah 53:3, Proverbs 18:21, 3 John 2, Psalm 91:14-16 (NLT). Numbers 23:19 (AMP) NKJV

RHEUMATIC FEVER

Before I ask You for anything, Father, I thank You for who You are. I thank You for all You have done and continue to do in my life. You deserve my worship, for You are the King of Glory. From the rising of the sun to its going down, Lord, Your name is to be praised.

I give thanks to You, Lord, for You are good! For Your mercy endures forever. For Your merciful kindness is great towards me, and the truth of the Lord endures forever. I will bless You, Lord, from this time forth and forevermore.

Praise the Lord! Before I call, You will answer; while I am still speaking, You will hear. I am seeking Your help from this inflammatory disease that is causing issues with my skin, joints, and heart. Father, Your Word states that whatever things I ask in prayer, believing, I will receive, and that if I can believe, all things are possible to me.

I have faith and trust in You that You can smother and release the inflammation in my joints. Strengthen my body from the fatigue; decrease and eliminate the pain in my chest and abdomen. Reduce and take away the fevers and strengthen my lungs and heart so that I won't continue to have shortness of breath. Decrease my enlarged heart and dissolve the fluid that is around it. I thank You, Father, for Your son Jesus and for allowing Him to take my infirmities and bear my sicknesses.

You have given me the keys of the kingdom of heaven and whatever I bind on earth will be bound in heaven; and whatever I loose on earth will be loosed in heaven. I bind up this inflammatory disease and ask that You kill it at the root. I loose total and complete healing in my body. So, I decree and declare my cardiovascular, skeletal, integumentary, respiratory, and nervous systems, along with my blood and immune system cells, will be in harmony with the design You established for their functionality.

According to Your Word, Jesus was wounded for my transgressions, He was bruised for my iniquities, and the chastisement of my peace was upon Him, and by His stripes, **I AM HEALED!**

Death and life are in the power of the tongue, so I speak life over my body. I decree and declare prosperity of healing over my body. In Jesus' name.

Whatever medication(s) I am prescribed, I pray that I will not get any side effects and it will help me, not further harm me, in the name of Jesus. Many are the afflictions of the righteous, but You, God, deliver me out of them all.

Thanks be unto You, who will give me the victory over this disease through my Lord Jesus Christ. I thank You that You will provide total and complete healing in my body. I wait for the Lord, my soul waits, and in Your word, I hope. Amen!

{Psalm 24:10, Psalm 113:3, Psalm 118:1, Psalm 117:2, Psalm 115:18, Isaiah 65:24, Matthew 21:22, Mark 9:23, Matthew 8:17, Matthew 16:19, Job 22:28, Isaiah 53:5, Proverbs 18:21, 3 John 2, Psalm 34:19, 1 Corinthians 15:57, Genesis 22:14, Psalm 130:5} NKJV

RHEUMATOID ARTHRITIS (RA)

Lord God of Israel, there is no God in heaven above or on earth below like You, who keeps Your covenant and mercy with Your servants, who walk before You with all their hearts. You are the only Wise God, through Jesus Christ, to whom be the glory forever. I give thanks to You, Lord, for You are good! For Your mercy endures forever.

You do great things and unsearchable, marvelous things without number. I will praise You first before asking for anything. I lift my eyes towards the hills from where my help comes. My help comes from the Lord, who made heaven and earth.

Thank You for allowing me to cast all my cares upon You, for You care for me. Father, I ask that You stretch forth Your loving hands and heal my fatigued and painful body. Smother and release the inflammation, loosen up the stiffness, and restore the strength in my joints. Protect the lining of my joints so RA will not cause erosion of my bones or deformity of my joints, Father.

I ask that You reverse my deformed hands and allow my fingers to be straight again. Slow down the progression and stop RA so it will not cause any further damage to my skin, lungs, heart, eyes, and/or circulatory system. If my circulatory system, eyes, lungs, and/or heart have not been impacted by RA, I ask that You protect them from having any involvement from RA. I pray to remain free from flare-ups, but should they arise, I ask, Father, that You minimize the length of the attacks.

I also pray that I not only go into remission but I stay in remission, and RA will not come upon me the second time. Allow me to go back to being pain-free and energetic again, Father. Have compassion on me, Lord, for I am weak. Heal me, Lord, for my bones are in agony.

You are the All-Knowing Physician who can heal and deliver me from this chronic inflammatory joint disease. I decree and declare my integumentary, respiratory, circulatory, nervous, musculoskeletal, and digestive systems, along with my blood and immune system cells, will be in harmony with the design You established for their functionality.

According to Your Word, Jesus was wounded for my transgressions, He was bruised for my iniquities, and the chastisement of my peace was upon Him, and by His stripes, **I AM HEALED!** Death and life are in the power of the tongue, so I speak life over my body. I decree and declare prosperity of healing over my body. In Jesus' name.

Whatever medication(s) I am prescribed, I pray that I will not get any side effects and it will help me, not further harm me, in the name of Jesus. Father, I believe You still perform miracles today. I ask that You perform one with me so RA will be a disease in the past for me. I thank You, Father, in advance for healing, deliverance, strength, and restoration in my body.

I ask that You turn my discomfort into comfort and allow me to live a full and healthy life. Thank You, Father God, that Your Word shall not return unto You void, but it shall accomplish what You please. For You are my Strength and my Song. I put my trust in You, Father. Amen!

{1 Kings 8:23, Romans 16:27 (AMP), 1 Chronicles 16:34, Job 5:9, Psalm 121:1-2, 1 Peter 5:17, Psalm 6:2 (NLT), Romans 11:33,

Matthew 9:12, Job 22:28, Isaiah 53:5, Proverbs 18:21, 3 John 2, Isaiah 55:11, Isaiah 12:2} NKJV

SARCOIDOSIS

Before I bring You my concerns, I want to give You praise and glory, Father.

You are worthy, O Lord, to receive glory and honor and power, for You created all things, and by Your will, they exist and were created. You are the Good Shepherd. The Good Shepherd who gives His life for the sheep.

Thank You for making me so wonderfully complex! Your workmanship is marvelous, how well I know it. The Spirit of God has made me, and the breath of the Almighty gives me life.

I am coming to You in labor and heavy laden. You promise when I come to You like this, You will give me rest. I ask for relief from the symptoms that I am experiencing from Sarcoidosis. Smother and release the inflammation in my lymph nodes, lungs, and/or skin. Give me energy and take away the fatigue.

Vanish the pain and strengthen my weakened joints and muscles, Father. **(Add any symptoms that you are having that are not listed.)** Shield my lungs, heart, and all other organs not impacted by this condition from harm. I seek Your healing for any other organs, ailments, or diseases that may be affecting my health.

Father, when I cry (for help), You will hear and rescue me from all the distress and troubles this condition is causing me. I decree and declare that my lymphatic, integumentary, musculoskeletal, urinary, circulatory, and respiratory systems, along with my blood and immune system cells, will be in harmony with the design You established for their functionality.

According to Your Word, Jesus was wounded for my transgressions, He was bruised for my iniquities, and the chastisement of my peace was upon Him, and by His stripes, **I AM HEALED!** Death and life are in the power of the tongue, so I speak life over my

body. I decree and declare prosperity of healing over my body. In Jesus' name.

Whatever medication(s) I am prescribed, I pray that I will not get any side effects and it will help me, not further harm me, in the name of Jesus. I will continue earnestly in prayer and be vigilant with thanksgiving. Thank you in advance for my healing shall spring forth speedily. You are All-Knowing and All-Powerful. I give You thanks always for all things, in the name of my Lord Jesus Christ. Amen!

{**Revelation 4:11, John 10:11, Psalm 139:14 (NLT), Job 33:4, Psalm 34:17,**

Isaiah 54:17, Matthew 11:28, Psalm 34:17 (AMP), Job 22:28, Isaiah 53:5, Proverbs 18:21, 3 John 2, Colossians 4:2, Isaiah 58:8a, Romans 11:33, Jeremiah 32:17, Ephesians 5:20} NKJV

SCHMIDT SYNDROME

Bless the Lord, O my soul! O Lord my God, You are very great: You are clothed with honor and majesty. I give thanks to You, Lord, for You are good! For Your mercy endures forever.

From the rising of the sun to its going down, Lord, Your name is to be praised. I praise You, Lord, for You are good; I sing praises to Your name, for it is pleasant. Before I call, You will answer; while I am still speaking, You will hear. Father, I come boldly to the throne of grace that I may obtain mercy and find grace to help in time of need.

I know that You are still performing miracles daily. I am calling on You, Father, to heal, deliver, strengthen, and restore my ailing body. My body has taken a hit due to the cluster of these three diseases. For type 1 diabetes, I ask that You regulate my blood glucose levels so they won't continue to fluctuate.

If there is anything I can do to help it on my end, like exercising and/or diet change, I ask that You give me the ability, strength and the dedication to do it. Take away the diabetes altogether so that I can stop taking these lifelong injections. Touch my thyroid and cause it to make enough thyroid hormones so that it won't be underactive. I don't want to have surgery and/or take radiation treatment, but if that is the way You will heal me, let Your will be done, Father.

Increase the production of my cortisol and aldosterone hormones so that it won't cause any damage to the adrenal cortex. I ask that You eliminate the pain, take away the fatigue, and strengthen my muscles/joints. **(Add any symptoms that you are having that are not listed.)** I decree and declare that my endocrine, urinary, and integumentary systems, along with my blood and immune system cells, will be in harmony with the design You established for their functionality.

According to Your Word, Jesus was wounded for my transgressions, He was bruised for my iniquities, and the chastisement of my peace was upon Him, and by His stripes, **I AM HEALED!** Death and life are in the power of the tongue, so I speak life over my body. I decree and declare prosperity of healing over my body. In Jesus' name.

Whatever medication(s) I am prescribed, I pray that I will not get any side effects and it will help me, not further harm me, in the name of Jesus. In my distress, I called upon You, Lord, and cried out to You; You heard my voice from Your temple, and my cry came before Your ears.

I want to thank You in advance for hearing my cry and rescuing me from the distress and troubles that this rare autoimmune disorder is causing me. Amen!

{Psalm 104:1, Psalm 106:1, Psalm 113:3, Psalm 135:3, Isaiah 65:24, Hebrews 4:16, Job 22:28, Isaiah 53:5, Proverbs 18:21, 3 John 2, Psalm 18:6, Psalm 34:17 (AMP)} NKJV

SCLERITIS

I give thanks to You, Lord, for You are good! For Your mercy endures forever. God, You are my strength; I will sing praises to You, For You are my Stronghold (my Refuge, my Protector, my Hightower), the God who shows me (steadfast) lovingkindness. I will praise the name of

God with a song and will magnify You with thanksgiving. Before I come to You with my cares, I had to give You praise first.

Father, I am casting all my cares [all my anxieties, all my worries, and all my concerns] once and for all on You, for You care about me [with deepest affection] and watch over me very carefully. Smother and release the inflammation in my eyes so that the symptoms of pain, tenderness, blurred vision, watery eyes, and severe sensitivity to light can go away, Father. If there is an underlying condition that I don't know that I have that has caused Scleritis, I ask that You let it be known. Give my physician and me wisdom, knowledge, and understanding of what it is and how it can be treated.

I pray that You will heal, strengthen, and restore my body from any sickness, disease, illness, or disorder, in Jesus' name. I decree and declare that my nervous system, along with my T-cells, blood, and immune system cells, will be in harmony with the design You established for their functionality.

According to Your Word, Jesus was wounded for my transgressions, He was bruised for my iniquities, and the chastisement of my peace was upon Him, and by His stripes, **I AM HEALED!** Death and life are in the power of the tongue, so I speak life over my body. I decree and declare prosperity of healing over my body. In Jesus' name.

Whatever medication(s) I am prescribed, I pray that I will not get any side effects and it will help me, not further harm me, in the name of Jesus. Thank You, Father, for hearing and answering my prayers. Every day, I bless You, and I will praise Your name forever and ever. Amen!

{Psalm 118:1, Psalm 59:17 (AMP), Psalm 69:30, 1 Peter 5:7 (AMP), Job 22:28, Isaiah 53:5, Proverbs 18:21, 3 John 2, Psalm 145:2,} NKJV

SCLERODERMA

Father, You are the Author and Finisher of my faith. The Everlasting

God, my Rock, and my Fortress. I give thanks unto You, Lord, for You are good! For Your mercy endures forever.

I open my lips and my mouth to show forth Your praise. Giving You honor and showing gratitude to You first is most important. I come boldly to the throne of grace that I may obtain mercy and find grace in my time of need. Father, I ask that You stop the overproduction of collagen in my connective tissue so that it will not cause any further skin or organ involvement.

Soften up my hard and tight skin and remove the calcium deposits so they will not cause any more damage to my skin and connective tissues. Having to endure the swelling and pain in my joints, muscles, and fingertips is not pleasant. There are times when I experience unbearable pain. Father, I ask that You eliminate the pain in my body so I don't have to continue to take these harsh pain medications that cause other problems in my body.

Smother and release the inflammation in my skin, fingers, joints, muscles, and esophagus. I ask for your divine protection over my heart, lungs, kidneys, and/or gastrointestinal tract, provided they are not compromised by this illness. If they have been impacted by this disease, I ask that You strengthen and heal each one of them. I know that weapons are going to be formed against me, but they will not prosper because I am protected by You, Father.

I decree and declare that my integumentary, cardiovascular, musculoskeletal, and respiratory systems, along with my blood and immune system cells, will be in harmony with the design You established for their functionality.

According to Your Word, Jesus was wounded for my transgressions, He was bruised for my iniquities, and the chastisement of my peace was upon Him, and by His stripes, **I AM HEALED!** Death and life are in the power of the tongue, so I speak life over my body. I decree and declare prosperity of healing over my body. In Jesus' name.

Whatever medication(s) I am prescribed, I pray that I will not get any side effects and it will help me, not further harm me, in the name of Jesus. I thank You that my healing shall spring forth speedily. I thank You in advance for restoring my health. You are my Strength and my Comforter. AMEN!

{Hebrews 12:2, Isaiah 40:28, Psalm 31:3, Psalm 107:1, Psalm 51:15, Hebrews 14:16, Isaiah 54:17, Job 22:28, Isaiah 53:5, Proverbs 18:21, 3 John 2, Isaiah 58:8a, Psalm 46:1, 2 Corinthians 1:3-4} NKJV

SJOGREN'S DISEASE

Father, You are the King of Glory. You are the Living Water that flows within me. You are the Lamb of God. You are a Consuming Fire.

I come before You with high praises in my mouth. I lift up my eyes to the hills from where my help comes. My help comes from the Lord, who made the heavens and the earth. You are the All-Knowing and All-Seeing God who knows how I am feeling and sees all that I go through with this prevalent autoimmune disease.

I thank Jesus for taking my infirmities and bearing my sicknesses. I stand on Your Word that whatever I ask for in prayer, believing, I will receive. I am believing for healing, deliverance, and restoration from this disease. Father, this dryness in my eyes, mouth, and vagina is not pleasant; neither are the other symptoms I'm experiencing from this disease.

I ask that You protect my normal exocrine glands from being attacked by my immune system. Touch my glands with Your healing hands, Father, so they can produce more moisture in my eyes, mouth, and other tissues so they will not cause further damage. This disease that I am being attacked with is not only causing me dryness, but it's also causing me to have brain fog, fatigue, chronic pain in my joints/muscles, swollen lymph nodes, heartburn, neuropathy, and kidney issues. I ask that You smother and release the inflammation in my joints and lymph nodes. Strengthen my weakened muscles and my memory. Give me energy like never before so that I can perform my daily activities and enjoy myself with family and friends without being fatigued.

For "Your grace is sufficient for me (Your loving kindness and

Your mercy are more than enough – always available – regardless of the situation); for (Your) power is being perfected (and is completed and shows itself most effectively in (my) weakness").

I decree and declare that my integumentary, digestive, nervous, musculoskeletal, reproductive, lymphatic, and immune systems, along with my blood and immune system cells, will be in harmony with the design You established for their functionality.

According to Your Word, Jesus was wounded for my transgressions, He was bruised for my iniquities, and the chastisement of my peace was upon Him, and by His stripes, **I AM HEALED!** Death and life are in the power of the tongue, so I speak life over my body. I decree and declare prosperity of healing over my body. In Jesus' name.

Whatever medication(s) I am prescribed, I pray that I will not get any side effects and it will help me, not further harm me, in the name of Jesus. I thank You, Father, that You are my physician, and my trust is in You for my healing. This hope (this confident assurance) I have as an anchor of the soul (it cannot slip, and it cannot break down under whatever pressure bears upon it)—a safe and steadfast hope that enters within the veil (of the heavenly temple, that most Holy Place in which the very presence of God dwells). Amen!

{Psalm 24:10, Jeremiah 2:13, John 1:29, Hebrews 12:29, Psalm 149:6, Psalm 121:1-2, Romans 11:33, Genesis 16:13, Matthew 8:17, Matthew 21:22, 2 Corinthians 12:9 AMP, Job 22:28, Isaiah 53:5, Proverbs 18:21, 3 John 2, Hebrews 6:19 AMP} NKJV

STIFF PERSON SYNDROME (SPS)

Father, I bring You my concerns after I give You the honor, praise, and glory that is due to You. You are The Most High God. You are the Lord who is there when I need You. You are the God who sees all that I am going through.

You are clothed with honor and majesty. Thank You for allowing me to bring You-my cares. For Your Word tells me to cast all my cares [all my anxieties, all my worries, and all my concerns], once and for all, on You, for You care about me [with deepest affection] and watch over me very carefully. Whatsoever things I ask in prayer, believing, I will receive.

Father, I ask that You heal, strengthen, and restore my body. I know that medication(s) and the physicians cannot heal me, but I know that You can, for You are my source of healing, Father. Protect my nervous system, especially my brain and spinal cord, from this rare progressive disease.

I ask that You take away the painful spasms that I have in my trunk and limbs, and cause me not to become mobility-impaired. Loosen and calm the stiffened muscles in my spine and lower extremities so that I will not wind up with a fractured bone. This is a lot on me mentally, Father. Therefore, I ask that You touch my mental state so my emotions will not cause the onset of spasms. Straighten up my spine if it's in any abnormal state, so that I will not become hunched over.

I decree and declare that my nervous, muscular, and endocrine systems, along with my central nervous system neurons and glial cells, will be in harmony with the design You established for their functionality.

According to Your Word, Jesus was wounded for my transgressions, He was bruised for my iniquities, and the chastisement of my peace was upon Him, and by His stripes, **I AM HEALED!** Death and life are in the power of the tongue, so I speak life over my body. I decree and declare prosperity of healing over my body. In Jesus' name.

Whatever medication(s) I am prescribed, I pray that I will not get any side effects and it will help me, not further harm me, in the name of Jesus. Thank You for being my Strength and my Strong Tower. Thank You for giving me peace, for You are the Prince of Peace. This attack on my body will not prosper, for many of the afflictions of the righteous, but the Lord will deliver me out of them all. Amen!

{Genesis 14:18-20, Ezekiel 48:35, Genesis 16:13, Psalm 104:1, 1 Peter 5:7 AMP, Matthew 21:22, Job 22:28, Isaiah 53:5, Proverbs 18:21, 3 John 2, Isaiah 12:2, Isaiah 9:6, Isaiah 54:17, Psalm 34:19} NKJV

SUSAC'S SYNDROME

Father, my mouth is filled with Your praise and Your glory all day long. When I need healing, You are my healer. When I need peace, You are my peace that transcends all understanding. When I am in pain, You are my painkiller.

I thank You for never leaving me nor forsaking me, Father. Before I come to You and bring You my concerns, I want to honor You, praise You, and give You glory. Your Word states that the effective, fervent prayer of the righteous man avails much. I have faith that You can and You will heal me from this rare autoimmune syndrome.

There is nothing too hard for You to accomplish. Touch my body with Your healing hands and heal my brain, eyes, and ears, Father. This disease is causing me to have headaches, difficulty walking, slurred speech, memory loss, and impaired vision. Father, take away the pain, strengthen my legs and mind, and correct my vision.

I thank You that You sent Your Word and healed me and delivered me from my destruction (my immune system attacking itself). I decree and declare that my nervous and muscular systems, along with my endothelial cells, will be in harmony with the design You established for their functionality.

According to Your Word, Jesus was wounded for my transgressions, He was bruised for my iniquities, and the chastisement of my peace was upon Him, and by His stripes, **I AM HEALED!** Death and life are in the power of the tongue, so I speak life over my body. I decree and declare prosperity of healing over my body. In Jesus' name.

Whatever medication(s) I am prescribed, I pray that I will not get any side effects and it will help me, not further harm me, in the name of Jesus. I thank You in advance, Father, for restoring my health and healing my wounds. Thank You for being my Restorer and a Good, Good Father. Amen!

{Psalm 71:8, Exodus 15:26, Judges 6:24, Philippians 4:7, Hebrews 13:5, James 5:16b, Jeremiah 32:17, Psalm 107:20, Job

22:28, Isaiah 53:5, Proverbs 18:21, 3 John 2, Jeremiah 30:17, Psalm 23:3} NKJV

SYMPATHETIC OPHTHALMIA (SO)

Father, You are the Creator. The Lord is There. You are the Most High God, and I sing praises to You. Holy and majestic are You, Father. Before I come to You with my concerns, I want to give You all the praise, glory, and honor that is due to You.

Lord, who made the heaven and earth. Bless You, Lord, O my soul! O Lord my God, You are very great: You are clothed with honor and majesty. I lift up my eyes to the hills from where my help comes from. My help comes from You, Lord, who made heaven and earth.

Thank You, Father, for allowing me to cast my cares upon You, for You care for me. When the righteous cry out (for help), Lord, You hear and rescue them from all their distress and troubles. Thank You for healing me from this vision-threatening eye disease. Father, I pray that You smother and release the inflammation in my eyes.

Reverse my blurred vision to clear vision so that it won't cause me to have visual impairment, which leads to blindness. I pray that You take away the pain, redness, and floaters in my eyes. You have healed all kinds of sicknesses and all kinds of diseases. I thank You that You don't have partiality, Lord; if You did it for them, I know You can do it for me.

I decree and declare my nervous system, along with my blood and immune system cells, will be in harmony with the design You established for their functionality.

According to Your Word, Jesus was wounded for my transgressions, He was bruised for my iniquities, and the chastisement of my peace was upon Him, and by His stripes, **I AM HEALED!** Death and life are in the power of the tongue, so I speak life over my body. I decree and declare prosperity of healing over my body. In Jesus' name.

Whatever medication(s) I am prescribed, I pray that I will not get any side effects and it will help me, not further harm me, in the name of Jesus. I thank You for restoring my eyes, Father. Thank You, Everlasting Father, for hearing and answering my prayers. Amen!

{Genesis 1:1, Ezekiel 48:35, Genesis 14:18-20, Psalm 104:1, Psalm 121:1-2, 1 Peter 5:7, Psalm 34:17, Romans 2:11, Matthew 4:23, Job 22:28, Isaiah 53:5, Proverbs 18:21, 3 John 2, Isaiah 9:6} NKJV

SYSTEMIC LUPUS ERYTHEMATOSUS (SLE)

Father, You are Beautiful Beyond Description. You are the All-Knowing God. You are the Rose of Sharon. You, O Lord, are a God full of compassion, gracious, long-suffering, and abundant in mercy and truth.

I want to give You honor, glory, and praise before I bring to You my concerns. Father, You made the heaven and the earth by Your great power and stretched out arm, and there is nothing too hard for You. I ask that You stretch Your healing hands towards me and heal me from this awful, chronic, long-lasting disease. This disease attacks my skin, joints, muscles, brain, kidneys, and arteries.

Father, You are my painkiller, and I ask that You take away the pain that I endure because of this disease. Smother and release the widespread inflammation in my body. Stop the tissue of my skin, joints, brain, kidneys, lungs, and blood vessels from being further damaged. Father, touch my body's immune system so it can stop fighting itself and causing a wreck in my body.

It is hard to do daily chores or work due to fatigue. Give me energy in my body so that I can get through the day. Take away fevers and stop them from forming, Father. I ask that You strengthen me mentally, Father, because going through this is tough and takes a toll on me.

There are some people out there with this same disease who want to commit suicide. I will not let that be me because my faith and trust lie in You, and I know that You can and will heal me. I appeal to You to prevent the individuals who are currently engaged in suicidal actions. Wrap Your loving and healing arms around them and let them know You love them.

Family and friends have abandoned me when I really needed them. Father, I thank You for not leaving me nor forsaking me. Before I call, You will answer, Lord, and while I'm still speaking, You will hear. So, I decree and declare that my cardiovascular, nervous, urinary, respiratory, musculoskeletal, and integumentary systems, along with my B cells, blood, and immune system cells, will be in harmony with the design You established for their functionality.

According to Your Word, Jesus was wounded for my transgressions, He was bruised for my iniquities, and the chastisement of my peace was upon Him, and by His stripes, **I AM HEALED!** Death and life are in the power of the tongue, so I speak life over my body. I decree and declare prosperity of healing over my body. In Jesus' name.

Whatever medication(s) I am prescribed, I pray that I will not get any side effects and it will help me, not further harm me, in the name of Jesus. I thank You in advance for healing, strength, deliverance, and restoration. You are not a man that should lie, nor a son of man that should repent. Have You not said, and will You not do? Or have You spoken, and will You not make it good? Your Word shall not return unto You void, but it shall accomplish what You please, Father. Thank You that my healing shall spring forth speedily. You are my Healer and my Deliverer. Amen!

{Romans 11:33, Song of Solomon 2:1, Psalm 86:15, Jeremiah 32:17, Hebrews 13:5, Isaiah 65:24, Job 22:28, Isaiah 53:5, Proverbs 18:21, 3 John 2, Numbers 23:19, Isaiah 55:11, Isaiah 58:8a, Exodus 15:26, Psalm 18:2} NKJV

TAKAYASU'S ARTERITIS

Father, You are The All-Sufficient One and the Lamb of God. You are my Shepherd and my Dwelling Place. I want to give You honor, glory, and praise before I bring to You, my concerns. Your Word states that I am Your masterpiece and am fearfully and wonderfully made.

I come boldly to the throne of grace so that I may obtain mercy and help in a time of need, for Your Word states that it's a good thing to quietly hope for help from God. Father, I cast my cares upon You concerning this chronic inflammatory autoimmune condition. I ask that You smother and release the inflammation in my blood vessels so that it will not cause damage to my organs and/or arteries.

For those in stage 1: Father, give me energy when I am fatigued. Cool my body down and take away the fever. You are my painkiller, Father, so please take away the pain in my muscles and joints. Touch me with Your healing hands and deliver me from this condition so that I won't progress to stage 2.

For those in stage 2: I'm crying out to You, Father, because my heart is overwhelmed due to the symptoms that I am experiencing. I ask that You stop the headaches, chest pain, dizziness, shortness of breath, and weakness in my limbs. Lower my blood pressure and stop the visual disturbances I am having. Touch me with Your healing hands and cause my healthy red blood cells to increase, delivering enough oxygen around my body. Also, cause me to no longer be anemic, Father.

Protect my memory from this condition. Stop the diarrhea. Father, stop the progression of this disorder so that it will not cause me to have a stroke or heart failure. I decree and declare that my circulatory, muscular, cardiovascular, nervous, respiratory, and digestive systems, along with my blood and immune system cells, will be in harmony with the design You established for their functionality.

According to Your Word, Jesus was wounded for my transgressions, He was bruised for my iniquities, and the chastisement of my peace was upon Him, and by His stripes, **I AM HEALED!** Death and life are in the power of the tongue, so I speak life over my body. I decree and declare prosperity of healing over my body. In Jesus' name.

Whatever medication(s) I am prescribed, I pray that I will not get any side effects and it will help me, not further harm me, in the name of Jesus. I thank You, Father, for healing, strength, deliverance, and restoration in my body. You are my Resting Place, and I find comfort in You. Amen!

{Genesis 17:1, John 1:29, Psalm 23:1, Psalm 90:1, Ephesians

2:10 (NLT), Psalm 139:14, Hebrews 4:16, Lamentations 3:26 (MSG), 1 Peter 5:7, Psalm

61:2, Job 22:28, Isaiah 53:5, Proverbs 18:21, 3 John 2, Jeremiah 50:6, 2 Corinthians 1:3-4} NKJV

TEMPORAL ARTERITIS/GIANT CELL ARTERITIS/HORTON'S DISEASE

Father, I want to give You the honor, glory, and praise before I bring You my concerns. You are the creator and beautiful beyond description. Holy, Holy, Holy are You, Lord; the whole earth is full of Your glory. I thank You for being the rock that is higher than me.

You are a Good Shepherd who understands and advocates on my behalf. Father, You said to put You in remembrance of Your Word. I thank You that Your Word shall not return unto You void, but it shall accomplish what You please. So, I come to You for help, asking that You hear and rescue me from all the distress and troubles that this disease is causing me.

This disease is causing me to have inflammation and damage to my blood vessels, which causes me to have fevers, fatigue, severe headaches, double vision, tenderness in my scalp, sudden loss of vision, unexpected weight loss, jaw pain, along with stiffness/pain in my shoulders, neck, and hips. Father, I pray that You heal, strengthen, deliver, and restore my body from this disease so that it won't cause me to have any further complications, including blindness, strokes, and/or aortic aneurysm. Smother the swelling, open up my blood vessels, and allow the blood to flow the way You made it to flow. Restore my oxygen and vital nutrients so that they will reach my body's tissues and cause the inflammation to go away.

I know that it is not my physician or the medication(s) that are going to heal me; it will be You because You are the source of healing. I have confidence in You that You will heal and restore my body, for You are the Restorer. So, I decree and declare that my circulatory, cardiovascular, nervous, skeletal, integumentary, and immune systems, along with CD4 T-cells, will be in harmony with the design You established for their functionality.

According to Your Word, Jesus was wounded for my transgressions, He was bruised for my iniquities, and the chastisement of my peace was upon Him, and by His stripes, **I AM HEALED!** Death and life are in the power of the tongue, so I speak life over my body. I decree and declare prosperity of healing over my body. In Jesus' name.

Whatever medication(s) I am prescribed, I pray that I will not get any side effects and it will help me, not further harm me, in the name of Jesus. Thank You, God, for being my strength and my shield; my heart is trusted in You, and I am helped; therefore, my heart greatly rejoices, and with my song I will praise You. Amen!

{Genesis 1:1, Job 9:10, Isaiah 6:3, Psalm 61:2, John 10:11, Proverbs 8:14, 1 John 2:1, Isaiah 43:26, Isaiah 55:11, Psalm 37:14(AMP), Jeremiah 30:17, Psalm 46:1, Job 22:28, Isaiah 53:5, Proverbs 18:21, 3 John 2, Psalm 28:7} NKJV

THYROID EYE DISEASE (TED)

Father, I give You thanks, for You are good! For Your mercy endures forever. You are the giver of life and my anchor. I want to give You the honor, glory, and praise before I bring You my concerns.

I am lifting my eyes to the hills from whence comes my help because my help comes from the Lord, who made the heaven and the earth. I am a child of God who is crying out for help. Your Word states that when the righteous cry (for help), You hear and rescue them from all their distress and troubles. Lord, I ask that You deliver me from this rare progressive autoimmune disease that is causing my body to mistakenly attack the healthy cells around my eyes, for Your Word tells me that Jesus heals all kinds of sicknesses and all kinds of diseases. Father, I ask that You take away my dry, gritty, redness, sensitivity to light, blurred/double vision, swelling, and pain/pressure in my eyes. I pray that You turn my bulging eyes back to the way You made them. I decree and declare that my endocrine, nervous, and immune systems, along with my orbital fibroblasts and immune cells, will be in harmony with the design You established for their functionality.

According to Your Word, Jesus was wounded for my transgressions, He was bruised for my iniquities, and the chastisement of my peace was upon Him, and by His stripes, **I AM HEALED!** Death and life are in the power of the tongue, so I speak life over my body. I decree and declare prosperity of healing over my body. In Jesus' name.

Whatever medication(s) I am prescribed, I pray that I will not get any side effects and it will help me, not further harm me, in the name of Jesus. I ask in faith without doubting that You heal me. Whatever things I ask in prayer, believing, I will receive according to Your Word. Thank You, God, for total healing and restoration. I thank You for being the Balm of Gilead and a miracle worker, Father God. Amen!

{Psalm 107:1, Job 33:4, Hebrews 6:19, Psalm 121:1-2, Romans 8:16, Psalm 34:17(AMP), Matthew 4:23, Isaiah 53:5, Proverbs 18:21, 3 John 2, James 1:6, Matthew 21:22, Jeremiah 8:22, Job 5:9} NKJV

TOLOSA-HUNT SYNDROME (THS)

Father, I will sing praises to You as long as I live and while I have my being. I give You the honor, glory, and praise for who You are. For I know You to be The Prince of Peace and The All-Sufficient One. Thank You for being The Way, The Truth, and The Life.

You gave me the right [the authority, the privilege] to become a child of God, that is, to those who believe in [adhere to, trust in, and rely on] Your name. Father, I cast all my cares [all my anxieties, all my worries, and all my concerns] upon You, for You care about me [with deepest affection] and watch over me carefully.

Father God, You are the source of healing. I know that You can heal me from eye pain, severe headaches, double vision, weakened muscles around the eye/face, eyelid drooping, and fatigue. I decree and declare that my nervous and immune systems, along with my lymphocyte and plasma cell infiltration, giant cell granulomas, and proliferation of fibroblasts, will be in harmony with the design You established for their functionality.

According to Your Word, Jesus was wounded for my transgressions, He was bruised for my iniquities, and the chastisement of my peace was upon Him, and by His stripes, **I AM HEALED!** Death and life are in the power of the tongue, so I speak life over my body. I decree and declare prosperity of healing over my body. In Jesus' name.

Whatever medication(s) I am prescribed, I pray that I will not get any side effects and it will help me, not further harm me, in the name of Jesus. I thank You in advance for healing me and answering an effective, fervent prayer of a righteous man/woman. After my healing, I will be able to testify that I overcame this by the Blood of the Lamb and the word of my testimony. You are my Strength and my Song. I love You, Father. Amen!

{Psalm 104:33, Isaiah 9:6, Genesis 17:1-3, John 14:6, John 1:12 (AMP), 1 Peter 5:7(AMP), Job 22:28, Isaiah 53:5, Proverbs 18:21, 3 John 2, James 5:16b, Revelation 12:11, Isaiah 12:2} NKJV

TRANSVERSE MYELITIS

Father, You are my Anchor, my High Tower, and my Day Spring. You are the Everlasting Father, the All-Powerful, so I give You the honor, the glory, and the praise, Father. I am Your masterpiece, and You have created me anew in Christ Jesus so I can do the good things You planned for me long ago. Before I call, You will answer, and while I am still speaking, You will hear Lord.

I lift up my eyes to the hills from whence comes my help. My help comes from You, Lord, who made heaven and earth. I bring before You this disorder that is causing me to have pain, abdominal sensations, urinary/bladder issues, weakness in arms/legs, and/or paralysis. I ask that You eliminate the pain, strengthen my body parts that are weak, smother and release the inflammation of my spinal cord, Father.

I thank You that Your grace is sufficient for me, for Your strength is made perfect in weakness. Most gladly, therefore, will I rather glory in my infirmities, that the power of Christ may rest upon me. Thank You, Father, for giving power to the weak and those who have no might; you increase strength. I thank You in advance for strength, healing, and restoration in my body.

I decree and declare that my nervous, musculoskeletal, and urinary systems, along with my neurons, endothelial, and glial cells, will be in harmony with the design You established for their functionality.

According to Your Word, Jesus was wounded for my transgressions, He was bruised for my iniquities, and the chastisement of my peace was upon Him, and by His stripes, **I AM HEALED!** Death and life are in the power of the tongue, so I speak life over my body. I decree and declare prosperity of healing over my body. In Jesus' name.

Whatever medication(s) I am prescribed, I pray that I will not have any side effects and it will help me, not further harm me, in the name of Jesus. Due to You healing and restoring my body, I can now tell others, look what the Lord has done! If He did it for me, I know that He can do it for You because He has no partiality. I thank You, Father, for delivering me from all my afflictions. Holy, Holy, Holy are You All-Powerful God. I thank You for being my Anchor. Amen!

{Hebrews 6:19, Psalm 144:2, Luke 1:78, Isaiah 9:6, Jeremiah 32:17,

Ephesians 2:10(NLT), Isaiah 65:24, Psalm 121:1-2, 2 Corinthians 12:9, Isaiah 40:29, Job 22:28, Isaiah 53:5, Proverbs 18:21, 3 John 2, Exodus 15:26, Psalm 18:2, Romans 2:11, Psalm 34:19, Jeremiah 32:17, Hebrews 6:19} NKJV

TYPE 1 DIABETES

Father, You are my Rock and my Fortress and my Deliverer; My God, my Strength, in whom I will trust; My Shield and the Horn of my Salvation, my Stronghold. The name of the Lord is a strong tower, and when I run to You, I am safe. Thank You for never leaving me nor forsaking me and for keeping me in perfect peace. As Your Word states, come to me all who labor and are heavy laden, and I will give you rest.

I lay at Your feet this Type 1 diabetes. I ask that You lower my blood sugar levels and allow my pancreas to make insulin so that my body will be rid of this autoimmune-related condition. Father, I acknowledge that this condition carries a substantial risk of major health concerns impacting my eyes, kidneys, gums, nerves, and heart. Please help me change my lifestyle, including my eating habits and physical exercise, so that it will prevent or delay any onset of complications.

Please minimize how much I have to urinate, as well as my eating and drinking intake. Clarify my vision and rejuvenate my energy, Father. I know that You are able to [carry out Your purpose and] do super abundantly more than all that we dare ask or think [infinitely beyond our greatest prayers, hopes, or dreams], according to Your power that is at work within us. Whatever things I ask in prayer, believing, I will receive.

So, I decree and declare that my urinary, endocrine, cardiovascular, nervous, and integumentary systems, along with my blood and immune system cells, will be in harmony with the design You established for their functionality.

According to Your Word, Jesus was wounded for my transgressions, He was bruised for my iniquities, and the chastisement of my peace was upon Him, and by His stripes, **I AM HEALED!** Death and life are in the power of the tongue, so I speak life over my body. I decree and declare prosperity of healing over my body. In Jesus' name.

Whatever medication(s) I am prescribed, I pray that I will not get any side effects and it will help me, not further harm me, in the name of Jesus. Thank You, God, that You are not a man, that You should lie, nor a son of man, that should repent. If You said it, You will do it. Thank You for healing, strength, and restoration. Amen!

{Psalm 18:2, Proverbs 18:10, Hebrews 13:5, Isaiah 26:3, Matthew 11:28, Ephesians 3:20 (AMP), Matthew 21:22, Job 22:28,

Isaiah 53:5, Proverbs 18:21, 3 John 2, Numbers 23:19(AMP)} NKJV

ULCERATIVE COLITIS (UC)

Father, I will praise the name of God with a song and will magnify Him with thanksgiving. You are the All-Sufficient One, Sovereign, and Self-Existing God. I love You, and I lift Your name. You are the Living Water and the Bread of Life. You show me the path of life; when I'm in Your presence, there is fullness of joy; at Your right hand are pleasures forevermore. I come boldly to the throne of grace that I may obtain mercy and find grace in a time of need.

Father, I ask that You minimize or eliminate the fatigue, bloody stool, loose/urgent bowel movements, abdominal cramps/pain, and persistent diarrhea. Smother and release the inflammation in my colon and eliminate the pain. No one knows how long I will have UC, but I do hear that people go into remission. Once I go into remission, Father, I pray that it will be permanent so that I can live a full and healthy life. Living with UC can be draining. I'm asking for strength because my body is weak.

Your Word states that You give power to the weak, and to those who have no might, You increase strength. I pray that You will provide my physician with wisdom, knowledge, and understanding of the best treatment for me. I decree and declare that my digestive system, along with my blood and immune system cells, will be in harmony with the design You established for their functionality.

According to Your Word, Jesus was wounded for my transgressions, He was bruised for my iniquities, and the chastisement of my peace was upon Him, and by His stripes, **I AM HEALED!** Death and life are in the power of the tongue, so I speak life over my body. I decree and declare prosperity of healing over my body. In Jesus' name.

Whatever medication(s) I am prescribed, I pray that I will not get any side effects and it will help me, not further harm me, in the name of Jesus. Thank You in advance that my healing shall spring forth speedily, Father. You sent Your Word and healed me, so I thank You, Father, for Your marvelous love, for Your miracle mercy to me whom You love. I trust in You, Lord [I commit myself to You, lean on You, hope confidently in You] forever; for You, Lord God, are an Everlasting Rock (the Rock of Ages). Amen!

{Psalm 69:30, Genesis 17:1-3, Genesis 14:18-20, Colossians 1:17, Jeremiah 2:13, John 6:35, Psalm 16:11, Hebrews 4:16, Isaiah 40:29, Job 22:28, Isaiah 53:5, Proverbs 18:21, 3 John 2, Isaiah 58:8a, Psalm 107:17-22 (AMP), Isaiah 26:4 (AMPC)} NKJV

UNDIFFERENTIATED CONNECTIVE TISSUE DISEASE (UCTD)

Father, who is like You among the gods, O Lord, glorious in holiness, awesome in splendor, performing great wonders. There is no other God besides You. You are worthy of my praise. You are my God, who has done for me these great and awesome things which my eyes have seen.

Father, You know how I have been feeling over the past few months. I have been struggling with this disease, along with the pain from it. After seeking help from the physician(s), I feel like there is no hope for me. It is disheartening to receive test results that confirm a lack of diagnosis, even though I am experiencing symptoms. When advised that there is no medical concern and that the pain is solely in one's mind, it raises the question of why such pain is being felt.

I am stressed out mentally, and I need Your help. I have had family members and friends turn their backs on me because they think I'm faking or it's all in my head. I'm not able to do the things I used to do because I don't have the strength or the energy. I feel like I'm mourning over my old self.

Your Word tells me to pray when I am suffering and sing songs when I am cheerful. Right now, I am suffering, and I need a touch from You, Lord. As Your Word states, to cast all my cares [all my anxieties, all my worries, and all my concerns], once and for all, on You, for You care about me [with deepest affection] and watch over me very carefully.

I come before You, asking that You smother and release the inflammation and eliminate the pain that I have been enduring. I decree and declare that my respiratory, cardiovascular, gastrointestinal, nervous, musculoskeletal, urinary, and integumentary systems, along with my blood and immune system cells, will be in harmony with the design You established for their functionality.

According to Your Word, Jesus was wounded for my transgressions, He was bruised for my iniquities, and the chastisement of my peace was upon Him, and by His stripes, **I AM HEALED!** Death and life are in the power of the tongue, so I speak life over my body. I decree and declare prosperity of healing over my body. In Jesus' name.

Whatever medication(s) I am prescribed, I pray that I will not get any side effects and it will help me, not further harm me, in the name of Jesus. I thank You in advance, Father, for renewing my strength, renewing my body, and regenerating my cells. Thanks be unto God, who gives me the victory through our Lord Jesus Christ. You are the Giver of Life, my Anchor, and my Everything Father. Thank You that Your Word shall not return unto You void but shall accomplish what You please. Amen!

{Exodus 15:11, Deuteronomy 32:39, Deuteronomy 10:21, James 5:13, 1 Peter 5:7 (AMP), Job 22:28, Isaiah 53:5, Proverbs 18:21, 3 John 2, 1 Corinthians 15:57, Job 33:4, Hebrews 6:19, Isaiah 55:11} NKJV

UVEITIS

Father, I give You thanks, for You are good! Your mercy endures forever. Blessed be Your glorious name, which is exalted above all blessings and praise! You do great things and unsearchable, marvelous things without number. You are a miracle worker. I lift my eyes to the hills from where my help comes. My help comes from You, Lord, who made the heavens and the earth.

Father, I come to You asking that You take away this inflammatory eye disease.

Smother and release the inflammation and eliminate the pain in my eye. Remove the redness and floaters from my eyes, clear up my blurred vision, and take away the sensitivity. Stretch forth Your healing hands towards me, Father, so that I will not have vital eye tissue damage that can lead to permanent vision loss. Whatever things I ask in prayer, believing, I will receive. I decree and declare that my visual, immune, and blood system cells will be in harmony with the design You established for their functionality.

According to Your Word, Jesus was wounded for my transgressions, He was bruised for my iniquities, and the chastisement of my peace was upon Him, and by His stripes, **I AM HEALED!** Death and life are in the power of the tongue, so I speak life over my body. I decree and declare prosperity of healing over my body. In Jesus' name.

Whatever medication(s) I am prescribed, I pray that I will not get any side effects and it will help me, not further harm me, in the name of Jesus. I thank You, Father, for hearing and answering my prayers. For Your Word states that the effective, fervent prayer of the righteous man avails much. I do not take seeing for granted, Father. I thank You for being the All-Powerful God and my Restorer. Amen!

{1 Chronicles 16:34, Nehemiah 9:5-6, Job 5:9, Psalm 121:1-2, Matthew 21:22, Job 22:28, Isaiah 53:5, Proverbs 18:21, Job 22:28, 3 John 2, James 5:16b, Jeremiah 32:17, Psalm 23:3} NKJV

VASCULITIS

Blessed are You, Lord God of Israel, our Father, forever and forever. Yours, O Lord, is the greatness, the power, the glory, the victory, and the majesty; for all that is in heaven and in earth is Yours; Yours is the Kingdom, O Lord, and You are exalted as head overall. Both riches and honor come from You, and You reign over all. In Your hand is power and might. In Your hand, it is to make great and to give strength to all.

Now, therefore, my God, I thank You and praise Your glorious name. Thank You for being my anchor and my deliverer, Father God. I come boldly to the throne of grace that I may obtain mercy and find help in time of need. Your Word states, "Come unto Me, all that labor and are heavy laden, and I will give you rest."

Father, I am casting all my cares (all my anxieties, all my worries, and all my concerns) on You, for You care about me. I pray, Father, for Your intervention to suppress and eradicate the inflammation of my blood vessels. Allow my blood to

Circulate without obstruction to prevent severe complications, such as damage to vital organs or the formation of aneurysms.

Father, do not turn away from me, the one who is suffering. Do not forget to help me while in pain. I thank You, Father, that the manifestation of my symptoms **[list all your symptoms]** from fatigue, fever, weight loss, and pain are no longer evident. Thank You that Your love and power surrounds me.

Thank You for helping me when I called and for answering my prayers concerning this disease. I decree and declare that my cardiovascular, digestive, nervous, skeletal, respiratory, and integumentary systems, along with my blood and immune system cells, will be in harmony with the design You established for their functionality.

According to Your Word, Jesus was wounded for my transgressions, He was bruised for my iniquities, and the chastisement of my peace was upon Him, and by His stripes, **I AM HEALED!** Death and life are in the power of the tongue, so I speak life over my body. I decree and declare prosperity of healing over my body. In Jesus' name.

Whatever medication(s) I am prescribed, I pray that I will not get any side effects and it will help me, not further harm me, in the name of Jesus. I put my trust in You, Everlasting Father. Amen!

{1 Chronicles 29:10-13, Hebrews 6:19, Psalm 18:2, Hebrews 4:16, Matthew 11:28, 1 Peter 5:7 (AMP), Psalm 22:24, Isaiah 53:5, Proverbs 18:21, 3 John 2, Proverbs 3:15, Isaiah 9:6} NKJV

VITILIGO

Father, You do great things, unsearchable, marvelous things without number. I will praise You, Lord, according to Your righteousness and sing praise to the name of the Lord Most High. You are the All-Knowing Physician who can heal and deliver me from this condition. In my distress, I called upon You, Lord, and cried out to You; You heard my voice from Your temple, and my cry came before You.

Father, this condition has caused my pigment-producing cells to die or stop functioning. Due to this condition, I am depressed, embarrassed, have low self-esteem, and want to isolate myself because of my appearance. There is no cure for this condition, and I do not want to be one of the ones who will have problems with my hearing and/or eyes, Father.

You are still performing miracles on a daily basis. I believe with all my heart that You can cure me from this condition, for Your Word states that You heal all kinds of sicknesses and all kinds of diseases. I pray that You restore, renew, remake, and regenerate my skin color, Father God. For You have made me wonderfully complex, and Your workmanship is marvelous. How well I know it.

I know when I am out and about, people stare, laugh, and/or talk about me because of my appearance. Help me to be strong and of good courage, and not fear nor be afraid of what people say about me. You are always with me and will not leave me nor forsake me. When I feel depressed, Father, I ask that You remind me that I am the apple of Your eye and hide me under the shadow of Your wings.

Father, You gave me the keys to the kingdom of Heaven, and whatever I bind on earth will be bound in Heaven, so I bind up depression, embarrassment, low self-esteem, and isolation. Whatever I loose on earth will be loosed in heaven, so I loose joy, happiness, confidence, and self-assurance. Father, I decree and declare that my immune and integumentary systems, along with my blood and immune system cells, will be in harmony with the design You established for their functionality.

According to Your Word, Jesus was wounded for my

transgressions, He was bruised for my iniquities, and the chastisement of my peace was upon Him, and by His stripes, **I AM HEALED!** Death and life are in the power of the tongue, so I speak life over my body. I decree and declare prosperity of healing over my body. In Jesus' name.

Whatever medication(s) I am prescribed, I pray that I will not get any side effects and it will help me, not further harm me, in the name of Jesus. Thank You in advance for healing, changing, and regenerating me, Father. You are the Giver of Life, my Healer, my Hiding Place, and my Comforter. Amen!

{Job 5:9, Psalm 7:17, Romans 11:33, Psalm 18:6, Matthew 4:23, Psalm 139:14 (NLT), Deuteronomy 31:6, Hebrews 13:5, Psalm 17:8, Matthew 16:9, Job 22:28, Isaiah 53:5, Proverbs 18:21, 3 John 2, Job 33:4, Exodus 15:26, Psalm 32:7, 2 Corinthians 1:3-4} NKJV

VOGT-KOYANAGI-HARADA (VKH)

I will praise You, O Lord, with my whole heart; I will tell of all Your marvelous works. I will be glad and rejoice in You; I will sing praise to Your name, O Most High. You show me the path of life; In Your presence is fullness of joy; at Your right hand are pleasures forevermore. Thank You in advance for healing and delivering me from this rare disorder.

Before I call, You will answer, and while I am still speaking, You will hear. Hear, O Lord, when I cry aloud; have mercy and be gracious to me and answer me. You stated in Your Word to seek Your face [inquire for and require Your presence as my vital need]. My heart says to You, Your face (Your presence), Lord, will I seek, inquire for, and require (of necessity and on the authority of Your Word).

Lord I am calling upon You, asking for help with this disorder. I have been experiencing eye pain, headaches, and dizziness. I pray that You will stretch forth Your healing hands and take away this disorder. I do not want to go into the next stage of this disorder and have hearing loss and inflammation in my eyes. Lord, I do not want to start developing vitiligo, alopecia, glaucoma, and cataracts. I ask that You smother and release the inflammation in my eye and eliminate the pain. Father, turn my discomfort into comfort and allow me to live a full and healthy life.

You gave me the keys of the kingdom of heaven, and whatever I bind on earth will be bound in heaven, and whatever I loose on earth will be loosed in heaven. I bind up all the symptoms that I have been experiencing and loose total healing, strength, deliverance, and restoration in my body. I decree and declare that my nervous, integumentary, and immune systems, along with my blood and immune system cells, will be in harmony with the design You established for their functionality.

According to Your Word, Jesus was wounded for my transgressions, He was bruised for my iniquities, and the chastisement of my peace was upon Him, and by His stripes, **I AM HEALED!** Death and life are in the power of the tongue, so I speak life over my body. I decree and declare prosperity of healing over my body. In Jesus' name.

Whatever medication(s) I am prescribed, I pray that I will not get any side effects and it will help me, not further harm me, in the name of Jesus. I thank You, God, that I am more than a conqueror, and I am already getting better. Thank You for allowing me to cast all my cares [all my anxieties, all my worries, and all my concerns], once and for all, on You, God, for You care about me [with deepest affection] and watch over me carefully. Amen!

{Psalm 9:1-2, Psalm 16:11, Psalm 18:2, Isaiah 65:24, Psalm 27:78 (AMPC), Psalm 50:15, Matthew 16:19, Job 22:28, Isaiah 53:5, Proverbs 18:21, 3 John 2, Romans 8:37, 1 Peter 5:7 (AMP)} NKJV

CONCLUSION (PRAYER OF SALVATION)

IN CONCLUSION, it is important to quote healing scriptures daily and speak life over your body. Do not let this illness dictate your identity or the person God intended you to be. You are a beautiful woman or handsome man, uniquely crafted, and God has a specific purpose for your life. As you take the 30-day challenge, add this affirmation to your daily healing scriptures: "I live like I'm living and not like I'm sick." Document your feelings before, during, and after the challenge, and express gratitude to God in anticipation of a positive outcome. Remember, warriors, you are not on this journey alone!

SALVATION

Salvation is a significant personal decision that each person must make independently, placing their faith in Jesus Christ. It means being saved from the consequences of being separated from God. This precious gift of eternal life is bestowed by God through the grace of Jesus. The Bible tells us that God loved the world so much that He gave His only Son so that anyone who believes in Him will not perish but will have everlasting life. Jesus suffered and died on the cross for our sins, was buried, and rose again to show His power over sin and death. If you're interested in receiving salvation or rededicating your life to Christ today, you can say this prayer.

SINNER'S PRAYER

If you would like to be saved, say this prayer.

I admit that I am a sinner, Father. I confess my faults to You, past, present, and future, and I turn from them all. I ask that You forgive me and cleanse me. Come into my heart, I accept Your son Jesus Christ as my Lord and Savior. Thank You for accepting me as a child of the Most High God.

Say these scriptures:

Romans 10:9-10

[9] That if thou shalt confess with thy mouth the Lord Jesus, and shalt believe in thine heart that God hath raised him from the dead, thou shalt be saved.

[10] For with the heart man believeth unto righteousness, and with the mouth, confession is made unto salvation.

Appendix A

Resources

Abdomen – Addison's Disease, Autoimmune Hepatitis, Bechet's Disease, Celiac Disease, Crohn's Disease, Endometriosis, Essential Mixed Cryoglobulinemia, Paroxysmal Nocturnal Hemoglobinuria, Polyarteritis Nodosa, Primary Sclerosing Cholangitis, Retroperitoneal Fibrosis, Ulcerative colitis

Arthritis – Juvenile Idiopathic Arthritis, Palindromic Rheumatism, Psoriasis, Psoriatic Arthritis, Reactive Arthritis, Rheumatoid Arthritis

Bile Ducts – Primary Biliary Cirrhosis, Primary Sclerosing Cholangitis

Bladder – Multiple sclerosis, Transverse Myelitis

Blood Clots – Antiphospholipid Antibody Syndrome, Immune Thrombocytopenia Purpura

Blood Vessels – Antiphospholipid Antibody Syndrome, Autoimmune Inner Ear Disease, Cogan's Syndrome, Crest Syndrome, Granulomatosis with Polyangiitis, Mixed Connective Tissue Disease, Polyarteritis Nodosa, Raynaud's Syndrome, Systemic Lupus Erythematosus, Takayasu's Arteritis, Temporal Arteritis/Giant Cell Arteritis/Horton's Disease, Type 1 Diabetes, Vasculitis

Bone Marrow – Pure Red Cell Aplasia

Brain – Balo` Disease, Guillain-Barré syndrome, Lupus, Mixcd Connective Tissue Disease, Multiple Sclerosis, Stiff Person Syndrome, Susac's Syndrome, Systemic Lupus Erythematosus

Cognitive Impairment – Multiple sclerosis

Colon – Ulcerative colitis

Ears – Autoimmune Inner Ear, Cogan's Syndrome, Relapsing Polychondritis, Susac's Syndrome, Vogt-Koyanagi-Harada

Eyes – Chronic Inflammatory Demyelinating Polyneuropathy, Cogan's Syndrome, Graves' Disease, Multiple sclerosis, Neuromyelitis Optica, Ocular Cicatricial Pemphigoid, Relapsing Polychondritis, Scleritis, Sjögren's Disease, Susac's Syndrome, Sympathetic Ophthalmia, Thyroid eye disease, Tolosa-Hunt syndrome, Type 1 Diabetes, Vogt-Koyanagi-Harada

Fatigue – Celiac Disease, Crohn's Disease, Granulomatosis with Polyangiitis, Juvenile Idiopathic Arthritis, Lupus, Myasthenia Gravis, Paroxysmal Nocturnal Hemoglobinuria, Polymyalgia Rheumatica, Primary Sclerosing Cholangitis, Psoriasis, Pure Red Cell Aplasia, Rheumatoid Arthritis, Sjögren's Disease, Vasculitis

Gastrointestinal – Crest Syndrome, Crohn's Disease, Endometriosis, Scleroderma, Sjögren's Disease, Undifferentiated Connective Tissue Disease, Undifferentiated Connective Tissue Disease,

Hair – Alopecia Areata, Discoid Lupus, Hashimoto's Thyroiditis

Headaches – Balo` Disease, Endometriosis, Paroxysmal Nocturnal Hemoglobinuria, Takayasu's Arteritis, Temporal Arteritis/Giant Cell Arteritis/Horton's Disease, Tolosa-Hunt syndrome

Heart – Lupus, Mixed Connective Tissue Disease, Rheumatic Fever, Scleroderma,

Hormone – POEMS (Polyneuropathy, Organomegaly, Endocrinopathy, Monoclonal Gammopathy, Skin Changes), Schmidt Syndrome

Joints – Addison's Disease, Ankylosing Spondylitis, Bechet's Disease, Crest Syndrome, Crohn's Disease, Essential Mixed

Cryoglobulinemia, Juvenile Idiopathic Arthritis, Lupus, Mixed Connective Tissue Disease, Palindromic Rheumatism, Polyarteritis Nodosa, Psoriasis, Psoriatic Arthritis, Reactive Arthritis, Rheumatic Fever, Rheumatoid Arthritis, Scleroderma, Systemic Lupus Erythematosus

Kidneys – Granulomatosis with Polyangiitis, IgA Nephropathy, Lupus, Mixed Connective Disease, Paroxysmal Nocturnal Hemoglobinuria, Retroperitoneal Fibrosis, Scleroderma, Sjögren's Disease, Systemic Lupus Erythematosus, Type 1 Diabetes

Liver – Autoimmune Hepatitis, POEMS (Polyneuropathy, Organomegaly, Endocrinopathy, Monoclonal Gammopathy, Skin Changes), Primary Biliary Cirrhosis, Primary Sclerosing Cholangitis

Lungs – Crest Syndrome, Granulomatosis with Polyangiitis, Lupus, Mixed Connective Tissue Disease, Sarcoidosis, Scleroderma, Systemic Lupus Erythematosus

Lymph Nodes – POEMS (Polyneuropathy, Organomegaly, Endocrinopathy, Monoclonal Gammopathy, Skin Changes), Sarcoidosis, Sjögren's Disease

Memory Loss – Lupus, Systemic Lupus Erythematosus

Muscles – Addison's Disease, Balo's Disease, Essential Mixed Cryoglobulinemia, Graves' Disease, Inclusion Body Myositis, Lambert-Eaton Myasthenic Syndrome, Lupus, Mixed Connective Tissue Disease, Myasthenia Gravis, Myositis, Undifferentiated Connective Tissue Disease, Polyarteritis Nodosa, Polymyalgia Rheumatica, Polymyositis, Scleroderma, Stiff Person Syndrome

Nerves – Balo`s Disease, Chronic Inflammatory Demyelinating Polyneuropathy, Endometriosis, Guillain-Barré syndrome, Lambert-Eaton Myasthenic Syndrome, Myasthenia Gravis, Parsonage-Turner

Syndrome, Tolosa-Hunt syndrome, Type 1 Diabetes, Undifferentiated
Connective Tissue Disease

Skin – Autoimmune Hepatitis, Bechet's Disease, Bullous Pemphigoid,
Celiac Disease, Crest Syndrome, Crohn's Disease, Dermatomyositis,
Discoid Lupus, Granulomatosis with Polyangiitis, Immune
Thrombocytopenia Purpura, Juvenile Idiopathic Arthritis, Lupus,
Mixed Connective Tissue Disease, Ocular Cicatricial Pemphigoid,
Pemphigus Vulgaris, Psoriasis, Psoriatic Arthritis, Pyoderma
Gangrenosum, Relapsing Polychondritis, Rheumatic Fever,
Sarcoidosis, Systemic Lupus Erythematosus, Vitiligo

Spine – Ankylosing Spondylitis, Balo` Disease, Psoriatic Arthritis,
Reactive Arthritis, Stiff Person Syndrome, Transverse Myelitis

Thyroid – Graves' Disease, Hashimoto's Thyroiditis, Schmidt
Syndrome

Urinary – IgA Nephropathy, Paroxysmal Nocturnal Hemoglobinuria

Appendix B

Healing Scriptures

Genesis 1:1 In the beginning, God created the heavens and the earth.

Genesis 2:4 This is the history of the heavens and the earth when they were created, in the day that the Lord God made the earth and the heavens.

Genesis 9:7 (NLT) Now be fruitful and multiply and repopulate the earth.

Genesis 16:13 Then she called the name of the Lord who spoke to her, You-Are-the-God-Who-Sees; for she said, "Have I also here seen Him who sees me?"

Genesis 17:1-3 When Abram was ninety-nine years old, the Lord appeared to Abram and said to him, "I *am* Almighty God; walk before Me and be blameless. ² And I will make My covenant between Me and you and will multiply you exceedingly." ³ Then Abram fell on his face, and God talked with him, saying:

Genesis 18:14 Is anything too hard for the Lord? At the time appointed, I will return unto thee, according to the time of life, and Sarah shall have a son.

Genesis 22:14 And Abraham called the name of the place, The-Lord-Will-Provide; as it is said *to* this day, "In the Mount of the Lord it shall be provided."

Genesis 35:3 Then let us arise and go up to Bethel; and I will make an altar there to God, who answered me in the day of my distress and has been with me in the way which I have gone."

Exodus 15:2 The LORD is my strength and song, And He has become my salvation; He is my God, and I will praise Him; My father's God, and I will exalt Him.

Exodus 15:11 Who is like you among the gods, O LORD, glorious in holiness, awesome in splendor, performing great wonders?

Exodus 15:26 And said, if thou wilt diligently hearken to the voice of the Lord thy God, and wilt do that which is right in his sight, and wilt give ear to His commandments, and keep all his statues, I will put none of these diseases upon thee, which I have brought upon the Egyptians: for I am the Lord that health thee.

Exodus 23:25-26 (MSG) But you-you serve your GOD, and he'll bless your food and your water. I'll get rid of the sickness among you; there won't be any miscarriages nor barren women in your land. I'll make sure you live full and complete lives.

Numbers 6:26 (NIV) The LORD turn his face toward you and give you peace.'"

Numbers 23:19 (AMP) God is not a man, that He should lie, Nor a son of man, that He should repent. Has He said, and will He not do? Or has He spoken, and will He not make it good?

Deuteronomy 7:9 Know therefore that the LORD your God is God; he is the faithful God, keeping his covenant of love to a thousand generations of those who love him and keep his commandments.

Deuteronomy 10:17 For the LORD your God is God of gods and Lord of lords, the great God, mighty and awesome, who shows no partiality and accepts no bribes.

Deuteronomy 10:21 He is your praise, and He is your God, who has done for you these great and awesome things which your eyes have seen.

Deuteronomy 28:13 And the Lord will make you the head and not the tail; you shall be above only and not beneath, if you heed the commandments of the Lord your God, which I command you today, and are careful to observe them.

Deuteronomy 31:6 Be strong and of good courage, do not fear nor be afraid of them; for the Lord your God, He is the One who goes with you. He will not leave you nor forsake you."

Deuteronomy 32:4 He is the Rock, His work is perfect; For all His ways are justice, A God of truth and without injustice; righteous and upright is He.

Deuteronomy 32:39 'Now see that I, even I, am He, And there is no God
besides Me; I kill, and I make alive; I wound, and I heal; Nor is there any who can deliver from My hand.

Judges 5:3 Hear, O kings! Give ear, O princes! I, even I, will sing to the Lord;
I will sing praise to the Lord God of Israel.

Judges 6:24 So Gideon built an altar there to the Lord, and called it [a]The-Lord-Is-Peace. To this day, it is still in Ophrah of the Abiezrites.

2 Samuel 22:4 I will call upon the LORD, who is worthy to be praised; So shall I be saved from my enemies.

2 Samuel 22:33 God is my strength and power, And He makes my way perfect.

2 Samuel 22:47 "The LORD lives! Blessed be my Rock! Let God be exalted, The Rock of my salvation!

1 Kings 8:22-23 Then Solomon stood before the altar of the LORD in the presence of all the assembly of Israel and spread out his hands toward heaven; **23** and he said: "LORD God of Israel, there is no God in heaven above or on earth below like You, who keep Your covenant and mercy with Your servants who walk before You with all their hearts.

2 Kings 20:5 "Return and tell Hezekiah, the leader of My people, 'Thus says the LORD, the God of David your father: "I have heard your prayer, I have seen your tears; surely, I will heal you. On the third day, you shall go up to the house of the LORD.

1 Chronicles 16:23-31 Sing to the LORD, all the earth; Proclaim the good news of His salvation from day to day. **24** Declare His glory among the nations,
His wonders among all peoples. **25** For the LORD is great and greatly to be praised;
He is also to be feared above all gods. **26** For all the gods of the peoples are idols,
But the LORD made the heavens. **27** Honor and majesty are before Him; Strength and gladness are in His place. **28** Give to the LORD, O families of the peoples, Give to the LORD glory and strength. **29** Give to the LORD the glory due His name; Bring an offering, and come before Him. Oh, worship the LORD in the beauty of holiness! **30** Tremble before Him, all the earth. The world also is firmly established, It shall not be moved. **31** Let the heavens rejoice, and let the earth be glad; and let them say among the nations, "The LORD reigns."

1 Chronicles 16:34 Oh, give thanks to the LORD, for *He* is good! For His mercy endures forever.

1 Chronicles 29:10-13 Therefore David blessed the LORD before all the assembly; and David said: "Blessed are You, LORD God of Israel, our Father, forever and ever. [11] Yours, O LORD, is the greatness, The power and the glory, The victory, and the majesty; For all that is in heaven and in earth is Yours; Yours is the kingdom, O LORD, and You are exalted as head over all. [12] Both riches and honor come from You, and You reign over all. In Your hand is power and might; In Your hand it is to make great And to give strength to all. [13] "Now therefore, our God, We thank You and praise Your glorious name.

Nehemiah 9:5-6 And the Levites, Jeshua, Kadmiel, Bani, Hashabniah, Sherebiah, Hodijah, Shebaniah, and Pethahiah, said: "Stand up and bless the LORD your God Forever and ever! "Blessed be Your glorious name, which is exalted above all blessing and praise! [6] You alone are the LORD; You have made heaven, The heaven of heavens, with all their host, The earth and everything on it, The seas and all that is in them, and You preserve them all. The host of heaven worships You.

Nehemiah 9:32 "Now therefore, our God, The great, the mighty, and awesome God, Who keeps covenant and mercy: Do not let all the trouble seem small before You That has come upon us, Our kings and our princes, Our priests and our prophets, Our fathers and on all Your people, From the days of the kings of Assyria until this day.

Job 5:9 Who does great things, and unsearchable, marvelous things without number.

Job 9:10 (AMP) Who does great things, [beyond understanding,] unfathomable,
Yes, marvelous *and* wondrous things without number.

Job 19:25 (AMP) For I know that my Redeemer and Vindicator lives, and at the last He will take His stand upon the earth.

Job 22:28 Thou shalt decree a thing, it shall be established unto thee, and the light shall shine upon thy ways.

Job 33:4 The Spirit of God has made me, and the breath of the Almighty gives me life.

Psalms 6:2 (NIV) Have mercy on me, Lord, for I am faint; heal me, Lord, for my bones are in agony.

Psalms 7:17 I will praise the Lord according to His righteousness and will sing praise to the name of the Lord Most High.

Psalms 8:4 What is man that You are mindful of him, And the son of man that You visit[a] him?

Psalms 9:1-2 I will praise You, O LORD, with my whole heart; I will tell of all Your marvelous works. [2] I will be glad and rejoice in You; I will sing praise to Your name, O Most High.

Psalms 16:11 You will show me the path of life; In Your presence is fullness of joy; at Your right hand are pleasures forevermore.

Psalms 17:8 Keep me as the apple of Your eye; Hide me under the shadow of Your wings.

Psalms 18:2 The Lord is my rock and my fortress and my deliverer; My God, my strength, in whom I will trust; My shield and the horn of my salvation, my stronghold.

Psalms 18:6 In my distress, I called upon the Lord and cried out to my God;
He heard my voice from His temple, and my cry came before
Him, even to His ears.

Psalms 18:30 As for God, His way is perfect; The word of the Lord is proven; He is a shield to all who trust in Him.

Psalms 21:13 Be exalted, O Lord, in Your own strength! We will sing and praise Your power.

Psalms 22:24 (Easy) God did not forget to help the man who was in pain. He did not turn away from the one who suffered. When he called to God for help, God answered his prayer.

Psalms 23:3 He restores my soul; He leads me in the paths of righteousness for His name's sake.

Psalms 28:6-7 Blessed be the LORD, because He has heard the voice of my supplications! ⁷The Lord is my strength and my shield; My heart trusts in Him, and I am helped. Therefore, my heart greatly rejoices, And with my song, I will praise Him.

Psalms 27:7 Hear, O Lord, when I cry with my voice! Have mercy also upon me and answer me.

Psalms 28:7 The Lord is my strength and my shield; my heart trusted in Him, and I am helped; Therefore, my heart greatly rejoices, and with my song, I will praise Him.

Psalms 29:1-2 Give unto the Lord, O you mighty ones, Give unto the Lord glory and strength. ²Give unto the Lord the glory due to His name; worship the Lord in the beauty of holiness.

Psalms 29:11 The Lord will give strength to His people;
The Lord will bless His people with peace.

Psalm 30:2 O Lord my God, I cried out to You, and You healed me.

Psalm 30:4 Sing praise to the Lord, you saints of His, and give thanks at the remembrance of His holy name.

Psalm 30:12 To the end that my glory may sing praise to You and not be silent. O Lord my God, I will give thanks to You forever.

Psalms 31:3 For You are my rock and my fortress; therefore, for Your name's sake, lead me and guide me.

Psalm 31:19 Oh, how great is Your goodness, which You have laid up for those who fear You, which You have prepared for those who trust in You in the presence of the sons of men!

Psalms 32:7 You are my hiding place; You shall preserve me from trouble;
You shall surround me with songs of deliverance. Selah

Psalm 33:1 Rejoice in the Lord, O you righteous! For praise from the upright is beautiful.

Psalms 34:1 I will bless the LORD at all times; His praise shall continually be in my mouth.

Psalms 34:1 (MSG) I bless God every chance I get; my lungs expand with his praise.

Psalms 34:17 (AMP) When the righteous cry {for help}, the Lord hears And rescues them from all their distress and troubles.

Psalms 34:19 Many are the afflictions of the righteous, But the Lord delivers him out of them all.

Psalm 35:27 Let them shout for joy and be glad, who favor my righteous cause; And let them say continually, "Let the LORD be magnified, who has pleasure in the prosperity of His servant."

Psalm 35:28 And my tongue shall speak of Your righteousness and of Your praise all the day long.

Psalms 39:7 And now, Lord, what do I wait for? My hope is in You.

Psalms 41:3 (MSG) Whenever we're sick and in bed, God becomes our nurse, nurses us back to health.

Psalms 41:3 (TLB) He nurses them when they are sick and soothes their pains and worries.

Psalms 46:1 God is our refuge and strength, a very present help in trouble.

Psalms 47:1 Oh, clap your hands, all you peoples! Shout to God with the voice of triumph!

Psalms 47:6-8 Sing praises to God, sing praises; sing praises to our King, sing praises. [7]For God is the King of all the earth; sing to him a psalm of praise. [8]God reigns over the nations; God is seated on his holy throne.

Psalms 48:10 According to Your name, O God, so is Your praise to the ends of the earth; Your right hand is full of righteousness.

Psalms 51:15 O Lord, open my lips, and my mouth shall show forth Your praise.

Psalms 54:6 I will freely sacrifice to You; I will praise Your name, O LORD, for it is good.

Psalms 57:2 I will cry out to God Most High, To God who performs all things for me.

Psalms 57:9-11 (AMP) I will praise and give thanks to You, O Lord, among the people; I will sing praises to You among the nations. [10]For Your faithfulness and lovingkindness are great, reaching to the heavens, and Your truth to the clouds. [11] Be exalted above the heavens, O God; Let Your glory and majesty be over all the earth.

Psalms 59:17 (AMP) To You, O God my strength, I will sing praises; For God is my stronghold {my refuge, my protector, my high tower}, the God who shows me {steadfast} lovingkindness.

Psalms 61:2 From the end of the earth I will cry to You, when my heart is overwhelmed; lead me to the rock that is higher than I.

Psalms 63:3-4 Because Your loving-kindness is better than life, my lips shall praise You. [4]Thus, I will bless You while I live; I will lift up my hands in Your name.

Psalms 66:1-4 Make a joyful shout to God, all the earth! [2] Sing out the honor of His name; Make His praise glorious. [3]Say to God, "How awesome are Your works! Through the greatness of Your power, Your enemies shall submit themselves to You. [4] All the earth shall worship You and sing praises to You; They shall sing praises *to* Your name." Selah

Psalms 68:19 (AMP) Blessed be the Lord, who bears our burden day by day, The God who is our salvation! Selah.

Psalms 69:30 I will praise the name of God with a song and will magnify Him with thanksgiving.

Psalms 69:34 Let heaven and earth praise Him, The seas and everything that moves in them.

Psalms 70:4 Let all those who seek You rejoice and be glad in You; And let those who love Your salvation say continually, "Let God be magnified!"

Psalms 71:8 Let my mouth be filled with Your praise and with Your glory all the day.

Psalms 71:14 But I will hope continually and will praise You yet more and more.

Psalms 72:18 Blessed be the LORD God, the God of Israel, Who only does wondrous things!

Psalms 73:26 (AMPC) My flesh and my heart may fail, but God is the Rock and firm Strength of my heart and my Portion forever.

Psalms 75:1 We give thanks *and* praise to You, O God, we give thanks, For Your {wonderful works declare that Your} name is near; People declare Your wonders.

Psalms 75:9 But I will declare forever, I will sing praises to the God of Jacob.

Psalms 86:10-12 (MSG) There's no one quite like you among the gods, O Lord, and nothing to compare with your works. All the nations you made are on their way, ready to give honor to you, O Lord, ready to put your beauty on display, parading your greatness, and the great things you do— God, you're the one, there's no one but you!

Psalms 86:15 But You, O Lord, are a God full of compassion, and gracious,
Longsuffering and abundant in mercy and truth.

Psalms 88:1 O Lord, God of my salvation, I have cried out day and night before You.

Psalms 90:1 (AMP) Lord, You have been our dwelling place [our refuge, our sanctuary, our stability] in all generations.

Psalms 92:1-2 (MSG) What a beautiful thing, God, to give thanks, to sing an anthem to you, the High God! To announce your love each daybreak, sing your faithful presence all through the night, accompanied by dulcimer and harp, the full-bodied music of strings.

Psalms 95:1-3 Oh come, let us sing to the Lord! Let us shout joyfully to the Rock of our salvation. ² Let us come before His presence with thanksgiving; Let us shout joyfully to Him with psalms.
³ For the Lord is the great God, And the great King above all gods.

Psalms 96:1 Oh, sing to the Lord a new song! Sing to the Lord, all the earth.

Psalms 96:4 (TLB) For the Lord is great beyond description and greatly to be praised. Worship only him among the gods!

Psalms 98:1 Oh, sing to the Lord a new song! For He has done marvelous things, His right hand and His holy arm have gained Him the victory.

Psalms 98:4 Shout joyfully to the Lord, all the earth; Break forth in song, rejoice, and sing praises.

Psalms 99:5 (AMP) Strong King, lover of justice, You laid things out fair and square; You set down the foundations in Jacob, Foundation stones of just and right ways. Honor God, our God; worship his rule! Holy. Yes, holy.

Psalms 99:9 Exalt the Lord our God, And worship at His holy hill; For the Lord our God is holy.

Psalms 100: 1-5 Make a joyful shout to the Lord, all you lands! ²Serve the Lord with gladness; Come before His presence with singing. ³Know that the Lord, He is God; It is He who has made us, and not we ourselves; We are His people and the sheep of His pasture. ⁴ Enter into His gates with thanksgiving, and into His courts with praise. Be thankful to Him and bless His name. ⁵ For the Lord is good; His mercy *is* everlasting, and His truth endures to all generations.

Psalms 102:1 Hear my prayer, O Lord, And let my cry come to You.

Psalms 103:1-3 Bless the Lord, O my soul; And all that is within me, bless His holy name! ² Bless the Lord, O my soul, And forget not all His benefits: ³Who forgives all your iniquities, Who heals all your diseases,

Psalms 104:1 Bless the Lord, O my soul! O Lord my God, You are very great:
You are clothed with honor and majesty,

Psalms 104:33 I will sing to the Lord as long as I live; I will sing praise to my God while I have my being.

Psalms 106:1 Praise the Lord! Oh, give thanks to the Lord, for He is good!
For His mercy endures forever.

Psalms 107:1 Oh, give thanks to the Lord, for He is good! For His mercy endures forever.

Psalms 107:17-22 (AMP) Fools, because of their rebellious way, And because of their sins, were afflicted. [18]They detested all kinds of food, And they drew near to the gates of death. [19]Then they cried out to the LORD in their trouble, And He saved them from their distresses. [20]He sent His word and healed them and rescued them from their destruction. [21]Let them give thanks to the LORD for His lovingkindness, And for His wonderful acts to the children of men! [22]And let them offer the sacrifices of thanksgiving and speak of His deeds with shouts of joy!

Psalms 107:20 He sent His word and healed them and delivered *them* from their destructions.

Psalms 107:21-22 (NLT) Let them praise the lord for His great love and for the wonderful things He has done for them. [22]Let them offer sacrifices of thanksgiving and sing joyfully about His glorious acts.

Psalms 111:1 Praise the LORD! I will praise the LORD with my whole heart in the assembly of the upright and in the congregation.

Psalms 111:3-5 His work is honorable and glorious, and His righteousness endures forever. [4] He has made His wonderful works to be remembered; The LORD is gracious and full of compassion. [5]He has given food to those who fear Him; He will ever be mindful of His covenant.

Psalms 113:3 From the rising of the sun to its going down, the LORD's name is to be praised.

Psalms 116:5 Gracious is the LORD, and righteous; Yes, our God is merciful.

Psalms 117:2 For His merciful kindness is great toward us, And the truth of the LORD endures forever. Praise the LORD!

Psalms 118:1 Oh, give thanks to the LORD, for He is good! For His mercy endures forever.

Psalms 118:17 I shall not die but live and declare the works of the Lord.

Psalms 118:28 You are my God, and I will praise You; You are my God, I will exalt You.

Psalms 119:147 (AMP) I rise before dawn and cry [in prayer] for help; I wait for Your word.

Psalms 119:169-176 (AMP) Let my [mournful] cry come before You, O LORD; Give me understanding [the ability to learn and a teachable heart] according to Your word [of promise]. ^{170} Let my supplication come before You;
Deliver me according to Your word. ^{171} Let my lips speak praise [with thanksgiving], For You teach me Your statutes. ^{172} Let my tongue sing [praise for the fulfillment] of Your
word, For all Your commandments are righteous. ^{173} Let Your hand be ready to help me, For I have chosen Your precepts. ^{174} I long for Your salvation, O LORD, And Your law is my delight. ^{175} Let my soul live that it may praise You, And let Your ordinances help me. ^{176} I have gone astray like a lost sheep;
Seek Your servant, for I do not forget Your commandments.

Psalms 121:1-2 I will lift up my eyes to the hills from whence comes my help? 2. My help comes from the Lord, who made heaven and earth.

Psalms 135:3 Praise the LORD, for the LORD is good; Sing praises to His name, for it is pleasant.

Psalms 139:14 I will praise You, for I am fearfully and wonderfully made; Marvelous are Your works, and that my soul knows very well.

Psalms 139:14 (NLT) Thank you for making me so wonderfully complex! Your workmanship is marvelous- how well I know it.

Psalms 144:2 My lovingkindness and my fortress, my High Tower and my Deliver, my Shield and the One in whom I take refuge, who subdues my people under me.

Psalms 144:9 I will sing a new song to You, O God; On a harp of ten strings, I will sing praises to You.

Psalms 145:1-2 (AMP) I will exalt You, my God, O King, and {with gratitude and submissive wonder} I will bless Your name forever and ever. [2]Every day I will bless You and lovingly praise You; yes, {with awe-inspired reverence} I will praise Your name forever and ever.

Psalms 145:3 Great is the LORD, and greatly to be praised; and His greatness is unsearchable.

Psalms 145:9 (MSG) GOD is good to one and all; everything he does is soaked through with grace.

Psalms 147:1 Praise the LORD! For it is good to sing praises to our God; For it is pleasant, and praise is beautiful.

Psalms 147:5 Great is our Lord, and mighty in power; His understanding is infinite.

Psalms 148:13 (KJV) Let them praise the name of the Lord, for His name is exalted; His glory is above the earth and heaven.

Psalms 149:6 Let the high praises of God be in their mouth, And a two-edged sword in their hand.

Psalms 150:2 Praise Him for His mighty acts; Praise Him according to His excellent greatness!

Psalms 150:6 Let everything that has breath praise the LORD. Praise the LORD!

Proverbs 3:5 Trust in the Lord with all thine heart and lean not unto thine own understanding.

Proverbs 3:8 It will be health to your flesh, And strength to your bones.

Proverbs 8:14 Counsel is mine, and sound wisdom;
I am understanding, I have strength.

Proverbs 12:25 Anxiety in the heart of man causes depression, but a good word makes it glad.

Proverbs 15:3 The eyes of the Lord are in every place, keeping watch on the evil and the good.

Proverbs 17:22 A merry heart does good, like medicine, but a broken spirit dries the bones.

Proverbs 18:10 The name of the Lord is a strong tower; the righteous run to it and are safe.

Proverbs 18:21 Death and life are in the power of the tongue, and those who love it will eat its fruit.

Isaiah 6:3 And one cried to another and said: "Holy, Holy, Holy is the Lord of hosts; The whole earth is full of His glory!"

Isaiah 9:6 For unto a Child is born, unto a Son is given; and the government will be upon His shoulder. And His name will be called Wonderful, Counselor, Mighty God, Everlasting Father, Prince of Peace.

Isaiah 12:2 Behold, God is my salvation, I will trust and not be afraid; For Yah, the Lord is my strength and song; He also has become my salvation.

Isaiah 25:1 O Lord, I will honor and praise your name, for you are my God. You do such wonderful things! You planned them long ago, and now you have accomplished them.

Isaiah 26:3-4 You will keep him in perfect peace, whose mind is stayed on You, because he trusts in You. [4] Trust in the LORD forever, for in YAH, the Lord, is everlasting strength.

Isaiah 40:28 Have you not known? Have you not heard? The Everlasting God, the Lord, the Creator of the ends of the earth, neither faints nor is weary. His understanding is unsearchable.

Isaiah 40:29 He gives power to the weak, and to those who have no might He increases strength.

Isaiah 40:31 But those who wait on the Lord shall renew their strength; they shall mount up with wings like eagles, they shall run and not be weary, they shall walk and not faint.

Isaiah 41:10 (AMP) Do not fear {anything}, for I am with you; Do not be afraid, for I am your God. I will strengthen you, be assured I will help you; I will certainly take hold of you with My righteous right hand {a hand of justice, of power, of victory, of salvation}.

Isaiah 43:15 I am the LORD, your Holy One, The Creator of Israel, your King."

Isaiah 43:26 Put Me in remembrance; Let us contend together; state your case, that you may be acquitted.

Isaiah 46:9 (MSG) "Think about this. Wrap your minds around it. This is serious business, rebels. Take it to heart. Remember your history, your long and rich history. I am GOD, the only God you've had or ever will have— incomparable, irreplaceable—From the very beginning telling you what the ending will be, All along letting you in on what is going to happen, Assuring you, 'I'm in this for the long haul, I'll do exactly what I set
out to do,' Calling that eagle, Cyrus, out of the east from a far country the man I chose to help me. I've said it, and I'll most
certainly do it. I've planned it, so it's as good as done.

Isaiah 53-5 Jesus was wounded for my transgressions, He was bruised for my iniquities; the chastisement of my peace was upon Him, and by His stripes I am healed.

Isaiah 54:17 No weapon formed against you shall prosper, and every tongue which rises against you in judgment you shall condemn. This is the heritage of the servants of the Lord, and their righteousness is from Me, says the Lord.

Isaiah 55:11 Your word shall not return unto You void, but it shall accomplish what You please.

Isaiah 58:8a Then your light shall break forth like the morning, your healing shall spring forth speedily.

Isaiah 64:8 But now, O Lord, You are our Father; we are the clay, and You, our potter; and all we are the work of Your hand.

Isaiah 65:24 (TLB) I will answer them before they even call to me. While they are still talking to me about their needs, I will go ahead and answer their prayers!

Jeremiah 2:13 For my people have committed two evils: they have forsaken Me, the fountain of living waters, and hewn themselves cisterns-broken cisterns that can hold no water.

Jeremiah 8:22 Is there no balm in Gilead, is there no physician there? Why then is there no recovery for the health of the daughter of my people?

Jeremiah 10:10 (MSG) But GOD is the real thing— the living God, the eternal King. When he's angry, Earth shakes. Yes, and the godless nations quake.

Jeremiah 17:14 Heal me, O LORD, and I shall be healed; Save me, and I shall be saved, For You *are* my praise.

Jeremiah 29:11 For I know the thoughts that I think toward you, says the LORD, thoughts of peace and not of evil, to give you a future and a hope.

Jeremiah 30:17 For I will restore health to you and heal you of your wounds' says the Lord....

Jeremiah 32:17 Ah, Lord God! Behold, You have made the heavens and the earth by Your great power and outstretched arm. There is nothing too hard for You.

Jeremiah 50:6 My people have been lost sheep. Their shepherds have led them astray; they have turned them away on the mountains. They have gone from mountain to hill; they have forgotten their resting place.

Lamentations 3:22-24 (AMP) It is because of
the LORD's lovingkindness that we are not consumed, Because His
[tender] compassions never fail. [23] They are new every morning;
Great *and* beyond measure is Your faithfulness. [24] "The LORD is my
portion *and* my inheritance," says my soul; "Therefore, I have hope in
Him *and* wait expectantly for Him."

Lamentations 3:26 (MSG) GOD proves to be good to the man who
passionately waits, to the woman who diligently seeks. It's a good
thing to quietly hope, quietly hope for help from GOD. It's a good thing
when you're young to stick it out through the hard times.

Ezekiel 48:35 All the way around shall be eighteen
thousand cubits; and the name of the city from that day shall
be: THE LORD IS THERE."

Daniel 2:20 Daniel answered and said: "Blessed be the name of God
forever and ever, For wisdom and might are His.

Daniel 4:34 And at the end of the time I, Nebuchadnezzar, lifted my
eyes to heaven, and my understanding returned to me; and I blessed the
Most High and praised and honored Him who lives forever: For His
dominion is an everlasting dominion, And His kingdom is from
generation to generation.

Nahum 1:7 The Lord is good, a stronghold in the day of trouble; and
He knows those who trust in Him.

Matthew 4:23 And Jesus went about all Galilee, teaching in their
synagogues, preaching the gospel of the kingdom, and healing all kinds
of sickness and all kinds of disease among the people.

Matthew 6:26 Look at the birds of the air, for they neither sow nor
reap nor gather into barns; yet your heavenly Father feeds them. Are
you not of more value than they?

Matthew 8:16-17 When evening had come, they brought to Him many who were demon-possessed. And He cast out the spirits with a word, and healed all who were sick, [17] that it might be fulfilled which was spoken by Isaiah the prophet, saying: "He Himself took our infirmities And bore our sicknesses."

Matthew 9:12 When Jesus heard that, He said to them, "Those who are well have no need of a physician, but those who are sick.

Matthew 11:28 Come unto me, all ye that labor and are heavy laden, and I will give you rest.

Matthew 12:28 But if I cast out demons by the Spirit of God, surely the kingdom of God has come upon you.

Matthew 16:19 And I will give you the keys of the kingdom of heaven, and whatever you bind on earth will be bound in heaven, and whatever you loose on earth will be loosed in heaven.

Matthew 17:20 So Jesus said to them, "Because of your unbelief; for assuredly, I say to you, if you have faith as a mustard seed, you will say to this mountain, 'Move from here to there,' and it will move; and nothing will be impossible for you.

Matthew 21:21-22 So Jesus answered and said to them, "Assuredly, I say to you, if you have faith and do not doubt, you will not only do what was done to the fig tree but also if you say to this mountain, 'Be removed and be cast into the sea,' it will be done. [22]And whatever things you ask in prayer, believing, you will receive.

Mark 1:34 Then He healed many who were sick with various diseases and cast out many demons; and He did not allow the demons to speak because they knew Him.

Mark 9:23 Jesus said to him, "If you can believe, all things *are* possible to him who believes.

Mark 11:23 For assuredly, I say to you, whoever says to this mountain, 'Be removed and be cast into the sea,' and does not doubt in his heart, but believes that those things he says will be done, he will have whatever he says.

Luke 1:37 (AMPC) For with God, nothing is ever impossible, and no word from God shall be without power or impossible of fulfillment.

Luke 1:78 Though the tender mercy of our God, with which the Dayspring from on high has visited us;

Luke 8:17 For nothing is secret that will not be revealed, nor anything hidden that will not be known and come to light.

Luke 10:19 God has given me the authority to trample on serpents and scorpions and over all the power of the enemy, and nothing shall by any means hurt me.

Luke 10:19 (AMPC) Behold! I have given you authority *and* power to trample upon serpents and scorpions, and [physical and mental strength and ability] over all the power that the enemy [possesses]; and nothing shall in any way harm you.

Luke 10:27 So he answered and said, "'You shall love the LORD your God with all your heart, with all your soul, with all your strength, and with all your mind,' and 'your neighbor as yourself.'"

John 1:29 The next day John saw Jesus coming toward him, and said, "Behold! The Lamb of God who takes away the sin of the world!

John 6:35 And Jesus saith to them, "I am the bread of life. He who comes to Me shall never hunger, and he who believes in Me shall never thirst.

John 10:10-11 The thief does not come except to steal, kill, and destroy. I have come that they may have life, and that they may have it more abundantly. [11]I am the good shepherd. The good shepherd gives His life for the sheep.

John 14:6 Jesus said to him, "I am the way, the truth, and the life. No one comes to the Father except through Me.

John 16:33 (AMP) I have told you these things, so that in Me you may have {perfect} peace. In the world, you have tribulation and distress and suffering, but be courageous {be confident, be undaunted, be filled with joy}; I have overcome the world. {My conquest is accomplished, My victory abiding}.

Romans 2:11 For there is no partiality with God.

Romans 8:16 The Spirit Himself bears witness with our spirit that we are children of God.

Romans 8:28 And we know that all things work together for good to those who love God, to those who are the called according to His purpose.

Romans 8:37 Yet in all these things we are more than conquerors through Him who loved us.

Romans 11:33 Oh, the depth of the riches both of the wisdom and knowledge of God! How unsearchable are His judgements and His ways past finding out!

Romans 16:20 And the God of peace will crush Satan under your feet shortly. The grace of our Lord Jesus Christ *be* with you. Amen.

Romans 16:27 To God, alone wise, *be* glory through Jesus Christ forever. Amen.

1 Corinthians 6:19 Or do you not know that your body is the temple of the Holy Spirit who is in you, whom you have from God, and you are not your own?

1 Corinthians 15:57 But thanks be to God, who gives us the victory through our Lord Jesus Christ.

2 Corinthians 1:3-4 Blessed be the God and Father of our Lord Jesus Christ, the Father of mercies and God of all comfort, [4]Who comforts us in all our tribulation, that we may be able to comfort those who are in any trouble, with the comfort with which we ourselves are comforted by God.

2 Corinthians 2:11 Lest Satan should take advantage of us; for we are not ignorant of his devices.

2 Corinthians 9:8 And God is able to make all grace abound toward you, that you, always having all sufficiency in all things, may have an abundance for every good work.

2 Corinthians 9:15 (AMP) Now thanks be to God for His indescribable gift [which is precious beyond words]!

2 Corinthians 12:9 And He said to me, "My grace is sufficient for you, for My strength is made perfect in weakness." Therefore, most gladly I will rather boast in my infirmities, that the power of Christ may rest upon me.

Ephesians 2:10 (NLT) For we are God's masterpiece. He has created us anew in Christ Jesus, so we can do the good things He planned for us long ago.

Ephesians 3:20 (AMP) Now to Him who is able to {carry out His purpose and} do superabundantly more than all that we dare ask or think {infinitely beyond our greatest prayers, hopes, or dreams}, according to His power that is at work within us.

Ephesians 5:20 Giving thanks always for all things to God the Father in the name of our Lord Jesus Christ.

Philippians 4:7 And the peace of God, which surpasses all understanding, will guard your hearts and minds through Christ Jesus.

Colossians 1:17 And He is before all things, and in Him all things consist.

Colossians 2:10 You are complete in Him, who is the head of all principality and power.

Colossians 4:2 Continue earnestly in prayer, being vigilant in it with thanksgiving.

1 Thessalonians 5:18 (AMP) In every situation {no matter what the circumstances} be thankful and continually give thanks to God; for this is the will of God for you in Christ Jesus.

1 Thessalonians 5:23-28 May God himself, the God who makes everything holy and whole, make you holy and whole, put you together —spirit, soul, and body—and keep you fit for the coming of our Master, Jesus Christ. The One who called you is completely dependable. If he said it, he'll do it! [25-27]Friends, keep up your prayers for us. Greet all the followers of Jesus there with a holy embrace. And make sure this letter gets read to all the brothers and sisters. Don't leave anyone out. [28]The amazing grace of Jesus Christ be with you!

1 Timothy 1:17 Now to the King eternal, immortal, invisible, to [a]God who alone is wise, be honor and glory forever and ever. Amen.

Hebrews 4:16 Let us therefore come boldly to the throne of grace, that we may obtain mercy and find grace to help in time of need.

Hebrews 6:19 The hope we have as an anchor of the soul, both sure and steadfast, and which enters the Presence behind the veil,

Hebrews 11:1 Now faith is the substance of things hoped for, the evidence of things not seen.

Hebrews 11:6 But without faith it is impossible to please him: for he that cometh to God must believe that he is and that he is a rewarder of them that diligently seek Him.

Hebrews 12:2 Looking unto Jesus, the author and finisher of *our* faith, who for the joy that was set before Him endured the cross, despising the shame, and has sat down at the right hand of the throne of God.

Hebrews 12:28-29 (AMP) Therefore, since we receive a kingdom which cannot be shaken, let us show gratitude, and offer to God pleasing service and acceptable worship with reverence and awe; [29]for our God is [indeed] a consuming fire.

Hebrews 13:5 Let your conversation be without covetousness; content with such things as ye have: for he hath said, I will never leave thee, nor forsake thee.

Hebrews 13:8 (AMP) Jesus Christ is {eternally changeless, always} the same yesterday and today and forever.

Hebrews 13:15 Therefore, by Him let us continually offer the sacrifice of praise to God, that is, the fruit of our lips, giving thanks to His name.

James 1:6 But let him ask in faith, with no doubting, for he who doubts is like a wave of the sea driven and tossed by the wind.

James 1:7 For let not that man suppose that he will receive anything from the Lord.

James 1:8 He is a double-minded man, unstable in all his ways.

James 5:13 Is anyone among you suffering? Let him pray. Is anyone cheerful? Let him sing psalms.

James 5:16b The effective, fervent prayer of a righteous man avails much.

1 Peter 5:7 Casting all your care upon Him; for He careth for you.

1 Peter 5:7 (AMP) Casting all your cares {all your anxieties, all your worries, and all your concerns, once and for all} on Him, for He cares about you {with deepest affection, and watches over you very carefully}.

1 John 2:1 My little children, these things I write to you, so that you may not sin. And if anyone sins, we have an Advocate with the Father, Jesus Christ the righteous.

1 John 4:4 You are of God, little children, and have overcome them because He who is in you is greater than he who is in the world.

1 John 5:4 (AMP) For everyone born of God is victorious and overcomes the world; and this is the victory that has conquered and overcome the world—our {continuing, persistent} faith {in Jesus the Son of God}.

3 John 2 Beloved, I wish above all things that you may prosper and be in health, even as thy soul prospereth.

Revelation 1:8 (MSG) The Master declares, "I'm A to Z. I'm The God Who Is, The God Who Was, and The God About To Arrive. I'm the Sovereign-Strong."

Revelation 4:8 (AMP) Holy, holy, holy {is the} Lord God, the Almighty {the Omnipotent, the Ruler of all}, who was and who is and who is to come {the unchanging, eternal God}.

Revelation 4:11 You are worthy, O Lord, To receive glory and honor and power; For You created all things, And by Your will they exist and were created."

Revelation 12:11 And they overcome him by the blood of the Lamb, and by the word of their testimony; and they did not love their lives unto death.

Revelation 15:3-4 (AMP) And they sang the song of Moses, the bondservant of God, and the song of the Lamb, saying, "Great and wonderful *and* awe-inspiring are Your works, O Lord God, the Almighty {the Omnipotent, the Ruler of all}; righteous and true are Your ways, O King of the nations! [4]"Who will not fear {reverently} and glorify Your name, O Lord {giving You honor and praise in worship}? For You alone are holy; for all the nations shall come and worship before You, For Your righteous acts {Your just decrees and judgments} have been revealed and displayed."

Revelation 19:11 Now I saw heaven opened, and behold a white horse. And He who sat on him was called Faithful and True, and in righteousness, He judges and makes war.

Revelation 19:16 And He has on His robe and on His thigh a name written: KING OF KINGS AND LORD OF LORDS.

Revelation 21:3-4 And I heard a loud voice from heaven saying, "Behold, the tabernacle of God *is* with men, and He will dwell with them, and they shall be His people. God Himself will be with them *and be* their God. [4]And God will wipe away every tear from their eyes; there shall be no more death, nor sorrow, nor crying. There shall be no more pain, for the former things have passed away."

Revelation 22:13 I am the Alpha and the Omega, *the* Beginning and *the* End, the First and the Last.

Revelation 22:16 I, Jesus, have sent My angel to testify to you these things in the churches. I am the Root and the Offspring of David, the Bright and Morning Star.

BIBLIOGRAPHY

- Aarda.org (Autoimmune Association)
- Aao.org (American Academy of Ophthalmology)
- Arthritis (CDC.gov/Arthritis)
- Arthritis.org (Arthritis Foundation)
- Autoimmuneregistry.org (The Autoimmune Registry)
- Autoimmuneinstitute.org (Global Autoimmune Institute)
- Celiac.org (Celiac Disease Foundation)
- Crohnscolitisfoundation.org (Crohn's Colitis Foundation)
- Aad.org (American Academy of Dentistry)
- Aad.org (American Academy of Dermatology Association)
- Dermnetnz.org (DermNet Dermatology Resource)
- Diabetes.org (American Diabetes Association)
- Endofound.org (Endometriosis Foundation of America)
- Enthealth.org (American Academy of Otolaryngology-Head and Neck)
- En.wikipedia.org (Wikipedia The Free Encyclopedia)
- Eyewiki.aa.org (American Academy of Ophthalmology)
- Healthline.com (Healthline)
- Liverfoundation.org (American Liver Foundation)
- Lung.org (American Lung Association)
- Lupus.org (Lupus Foundation of America)
- Lupus Survivor Incorporated Lupussurvivorgroup@gmail.com Facebook.com/lupussurvivorinc
- Mayoclinic.org (Mayo Clinic)
- Mda.org (Muscular Dystrophy Association)
- Medlineplus.gov (Medline Plus National Library of Medicine)
- Merckmanuals.com (Merck Manuals)
- My.Clevelandclinic.org (Cleveland Clinic)
- Myositis.org (Myositis Association)
- Nationalmssociety.org (National Multiple Sclerosis Society)
- Niams.nih.gov (National Institute of Arthritis and Musculoskeletal and Skin Disease)
- Nhlbi.nih.gov (National Institutes of Health)
- Pubmed.ncbi.nlm.nih.gov (National Center for Biotechnology Information)
- Raredisease.org (National Organization for Rare Diseases)
- Rheumatology.org (American College of Rheumatology)

BIBLIOGRAPHY

- Spondylitis.org (Spondylitis Association of America)
- Stopsarcoidosis.org (Foundation for Sarcoidosis Research)
- Thyroid.org (American Thyroid Association)
- Uptodate.com (Solutions Up To Date/Wolters Kluwer)
- Vasculitisfoundation.org (Vasculitis Foundation)
- Verywellhealth.com (Very Well Health – Health Information)
- Wedmd.com (Web MD)
- The Weapons of our Warfare (Kenneth Scott)

ABOUT THE AUTHOR

Nikita Thompson is a woman of faith, wife, mother, and business owner. She was born and raised in Newark, New Jersey, where she met her high school sweetheart and now husband of 30-plus years, Larry Thompson. They share two beautiful children together, DaVante' Thompson and De'Ja Caldwell. They wanted a better life for their children, so they moved to Georgia and then relocated to the sunny suburbs of Florida. Little did Nikita know this move would be more than just beneficial for her children, but also for her health.

Her first-ever rheumatologist diagnosed her with Raynaud's disease, systemic lupus, and then mixed connective tissue disease. She went through a season of depression and loneliness, but continued to be an amazing wife and loving mother.

Even though she was unable to work any longer, God still had plans for Nikita.

In 2018, she created the 501(c) Lupus Survivors Incorporation Support Group.

Her mission for this group is to show empathy, empowerment, comfort, and aid financially and emotionally to those living with any autoimmune disorder. Nikita is the epitome of turning pain into purpose. She is an inspiration to those around her to keep fighting, no matter the obstacles we may face. She has proven time and time again that tears are not a sign that faith or hope in God has been lost; it is a sign that we can feel the pain while declaring God's Word.

" I shall not die, but live, And declare the works of the LORD."
Psalm 118:17 KJV

"This is the day which the Lord hath made; we will rejoice and be glad in it." Psalm 118:24 KJV

www.ingramcontent.com/pod-product-compliance
Lightning Source LLC
Chambersburg PA
CBHW072145270326
41931CB00010B/1889